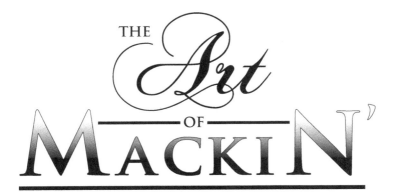

2009
G.D Publishing
King Flex Entertainment

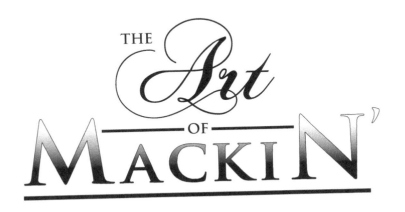

THE Art OF MACKIN'

BY
TARIQ "KING FLEX" NASHEED

FOREWORD

When I first began writing The Art Of Mackin' during the months of July through November of 1999, I had one main goal in mind; *talk about dating and relationships from a real man's perspective.* I wanted to break down the raw truths of the dating /mackin' game without having to hide behind the shadows of political correctness.

When the book was finally released the following year, for a brief period of time, some media outlets treated me like the anti-Christ. Certain people in television, radio, magazines and feminist groups, etc. were up in arms:"*How dare this guy write a book teaching men such despicable things as being a player, a womanizer and a mack.* "

These were some of the things said about me during the first few months of the initial release of The Art Of Mackin'. Once people got over the title and the misperception of what they thought "mackin" was, there was a collective change of opinion about the book. They learned that mackin'- true mackin' that is- is really about manhood and integrity.

As I hope you learn by reading this book, mackin', manhood and integrity can transcend just man-woman relationships. It can be applied to all other aspects of life

Tariq "King Flex" Nasheed

TABLE OF CONTENTS

INTRODUCTION

This book, The Art of Mackin', takes a unique, yet serious look at modern male/female relationships from a player's point of view. Currently, there are many relationship books geared towards women ("The Rules," "How to Marry a Man," etc.) that teach women how to subtly manipulate men into relationships.

The Art of Mackin' is the first how-to book that teaches men how to actually become true players and macks and how to use certain techniques (not deceit) in order to get what they want from women. Whether it is sex, money or companionship, this book teaches men what to say, verbatim, in order to reach their intended goal. By using these techniques, I am not implying that you do anything negative. I am just teaching guys to stay on top of their game when dealing with women.

The Art of Mackin' is also the first book that tells men what to say, word for word, in order to get sex from women, guaranteed. By using my tried and proven methods of mackin', men are guaranteed to increase their player ratio by at least fifty percent (50%).

The information in this book is intended for women to read as well. By soaking in some of this game, women can take an objective look at themselves, and touch up on *their* skills. Women will see a little bit of themselves in some of the females I describe throughout the chapters. I give full descriptions and details of all types of women, ranging from top-notch women, to independent women, hoodrats, chickenheads, groupies, hoochies, hookers, and everything else in between.

Many women have asked me questions such as, "Why are you writing a book showing men how to be macks and players?" And they have said things like, "That's the problem now. We have too many men that are trying to be players and not enough responsible men."

One thing that I have noticed is that most of the women who say this are players themselves, and they don't want a guy they are dealing with to learn game, because then they won't be able to get over on him anymore. The fact of the matter is many females are better players than men , because women are better at being manipulative and cunning. Women who are players screen for guys who have no game, because they can then manipulate them for their own benefit.

Don't get me wrong. There are many Top notch women out there who have themselves together and who would make excellent mates. But a top notch female is like a diamond, and in order to get a diamond, you have to dig and search in all the right places. The problem is that we have too many "cubic zirconium" females walking around on the surface that are easily accessible.

One of the purposes of this book is to help men sift through the fake females to get to the diamond girls. (This screening process is especially needed here in L.A. where many people feel that it is a necessity to put up a front. Since the concept of Hollywood is built on an image, many people come here thinking that they have to enter into that image 24/7. This is why so many people get caught up trying to live the proverbial L.A. life, because they fail to realize that "Hollywood" is a job, not a lifestyle.) Unfortunately, since many cubic zirconium females tend to stand out and receive so much attention, people get the assumption that most are like this, and obviously that is not true.

This is why it's important for a man to know how to peep game when dealing with women. I could tell all men to go out and get the first good woman you see, settle down, and live happily ever after. But, for the most part, this is unrealistic thinking, because if it were that simple the world would be a better place. You have to have at least some level of game evaluation to figure out which females are good for you, and which ones are not. If you don't have game, you could be in a relationship thinking you have a good woman when you really have an undercover hood rat or trailor chick.

Now, if you are a guy who is in a relationship, and you know without a shadow of a doubt that you have a down female, by all means continue to maintain that relationship. You should utilize some of the information in this book to keep up the level of intrigue within the boundaries of your relationship. But if you are a single man, this book should be used as your reference guide from this point on (or at least until you settle down).

Also, by writing this book, I intend to give people a voyeuristic view into the life of a player and a mack. I want to give people an idea of how a mack thinks and evaluates women. I also hope to clear up some of the myths and misconceptions that surround macks and players.

As I mentioned before, even though I have made many humorous observations throughout the chapters, the contents in this book are very serious, and they are extremely effective. A lot of this information will benefit women directly and indirectly, because I give men tips on elevating themselves (verbally and sexually) which, in turn, helps them satisfy women better.

Reading this book will help men to:
*Overcome the fear of getting dissed by women and help boost their confidence.

*Approach women more smoothly and correctly.

*Learn ways to stimulate women mentally and physically.

*Improve (and increase) their sex lives.

*Lift their self-esteem, which in turn, makes them more desirable to women.

Now, some of the language and terminology throughout this book may seem borderline misogynistic, but in order to give you a clear idea of what goes on in the mind of a mack, and how the game is put down, I have to use certain street euphemisms and player colloquialisms. The main misconception about the mackin' game is that many men feel they have to step to women with lies and deception in order to get any play. The number one rule of being a successful mack is to *be true to the game, and the game will be true to you*. Although a few white lies are fair game for an aspiring mack or player, a truly seasoned mack's game should be so tight, he should have no problem coming across as honest as possible. If a person has become accustomed to deceiving others, after a period of time that person will start deceiving himself. This, in turn, creates circular reasoning. When people go into relationships with deceitful intentions, they often have the nerve to get frustrated when the outcome of the relationships is negative. For example, a guy might say to himself "I can't get a woman unless I'm flossin or high rollin'." So he goes out and purchases flamboyant clothes, glitzy jewelry, and tries to entice women by flashing his cash and claming that he can do all sorts of extravagant things for them. Then, when certain females call his bluff and drain his bank account dry, he complains that, "All these females just want money" and "Why can't I find a woman who wants me for me?" He went full circle by creating a negative scenario, and then becoming disappointed by the negative outcome.

Many females will say to themselves, "If I show off my body, I can get more attention from men." So they start dressing hoochie. They then have the nerve to claim that, "All men want is sex. Why can't I find a man who likes me for the person I am inside? Why can't I find a good man?" These women never think to ask themselves, why would a good man want a hoochie? This is why it is very important to be true to yourself and true to the game.

Some of the most common questions that people ask me are: "What makes you, Tariq, such an expert on the art of mackin'? Are you still a player? If not, what made you stop? How did you learn all this 'game'? Since you have so much game, can you get any woman you want?"

Many people "mack" for recreational purposes, but I was at a point in my life where I had to mack out of necessity. During my teenage years, I was living on my own out here in Los Angeles, and this brought on a certain level of responsibility. Since I didn't have any other adequate skills to aid in my survival and standard of living, I had to utilize the resources that were given to me naturally. Those resources were hustlin' and mackin'. The essence of mackin' is having the power of persuasion. 1

figured that a person who is charismatic and persuasive can achieve anything they want in life, and this is what made me become very thorough with my game. By me having dealt with thousands of women over the years, I've basically learned the art of mackin' from a hands-on, trial and error approach.

But, I have volunteerily turned in my player card. Most players get out of the game because of old age. They reach a certain point in their lives where they run out of options when it comes to females, so they then decide to settle down and get married. Basically, many players get *forced* into retirement. This wasn't the case with me, because I still have the option to be in the game. The reason I'm not in the game anymore is because I've mastered the game, and what fun is it to play a game when you already know the outcome? When you become an expert on peeping game and figuring females out, it is no longer a challenge for you to play the field. So, basically, I'm no longer a *player,* I'm now a *coach.*

Most men start to perfect their mackin' skills in their late 20's and early 30's. Normally, when a man is in his late teens/early 20 's, he may be going to school, just starting a new career, etc., and his money isn't right at this point.

This somewhat limits his dating options. Many brothers at this age tend to date the local little hoodrats that are in his immediate community. But when a guy reaches his late 20's, he becomes more financially stable, and he now has the means to step up his lifestyle. He is now able to maintain a decent car and a decent home, and he is also able to branch out and date a variety of different females from all walks of life. And the more options you have, the more experience you can gain.

Many men feel they need about six or seven years of playing the field or getting their mack on. So many men start dwindling out of their player stage when they reach their mid- to late 30's. Once a man grows tired of playing the field, he becomes more relaxed in his demeanor, and more honest with himself and the females he deals with. This is why women say that men are the most sexy at around age 40.

From my early teens, I moved around a lot, from city to city, and this exposed me to a variety of types of females. Since I had more responsibilities than the average person my age, I was able to attract a class of females that were more socially advanced. Experiencing this better class of women put me in the position to tighten up my game at an early age. Consequently, I was able to grow out of my player stage at a relatively early age as well. Since I'm not in "the game" anymore, I don't have a problem with sharing some of my mackin' secrets and tricks of the trade. Being a mack doesn't mean that you can get any woman you want. No one can get anybody they want. That's just not reality, because every woman has different tastes. If you are a Black man who wants to get with a female who only dates Eskimos, you're wasting your time, because if you can't build her an igloo, she's not going to give you the time of day. That doesn't mean that anything is wrong with you, it's just that the female has a fetish for something totally different. So the mackin' game is about screening for women who want you as much as you want them. There's an old saying that states, "There is someone for everybody," and that saying is extremely true. Plus, it's foolish to want someone who doesn't want you anyway. No matter how you look, or what your situation is, every brother has mackin' potential. If you have the confidence to put the mack down and make yourself available for women to soak in your game, you should have no problems satisfying your relationship agendas. (One of the rules of the game is that you have to sometimes have a slot machine mentality: If you keep on playing the "slots," you're bound to hit a jackpot sooner or later.)

I have a friend who was in a car accident many years ago, and it knocked out most of his teeth and slightly disfigured his nose. And even with his disfigurements, my friend still has a different female at his crib every night. Why? Because he knows how to put his bid in. He keeps fishing for females until one of them takes the bait. Plus, he has become totally immune to getting dissed. He also understands that one woman's frog is another woman's prince. So, for every ten females who kick him to the curb, there are going to be two females who will catch him. This is why you have to make yourself available for women to peep you out. Sitting around at home, afraid to get out because you might get dissed, is simply not going to cut it. You have to at least put yourself in a position to socialize with women. Even if you just like hangin' out with your boys, gather up your homies and hang out where females hang out (and I don't mean strip clubs).

Even if you're not spitting game when you go out, there's still a chance for you to come up. I remember I used to see this one brother at all the clubs throughout Los Angeles. He was a normal-looking brother, but he had one leg. One of my female friends, who used to always see him at the clubs as well, said to me, "You know, I kinda feel sorry for that guy with the one leg. 1 see him everywhere I go. I bet females don't give him the time of day. Well, I know what," she continued, "I'm gonna help that brother out. I'm gonna give him some ass. Plus, I've never done it with a brother with one leg before, so it might be kinda freaky." (And this is a nice looking female, mind you.) The point is, if this brother just sat around worrying about getting dissed, he would have missed out on a pleasurable opportunity. He got out and made himself available to women, like a mack is supposed to do. Sure, the female had sex with him out of sympathy, but there is nothing wrong with a little "pity pussy."

Another important thing to know about being a mack is that you must have a lot of *self discipline*. This is important, so that you won't have a need to hound women for sex. A lack of control over his sexual desires has been man's downfall since the beginning of time (as in the case of Samson and Delilah, Anthony and Cleopatra, Jim Baker and Jessica Hahn, Bill Clinton and Monica, etc.). There is no way for a man to become a successful mack unless he learns how to control his sexual appetite. (One way to learn self-discipline is to fast. If you can control something as natural as eating, then you can control anything.) Once you gain control over your sexual libido, you will learn to make decisions with your *big head* instead of your *dick head*.

I must also note that there is a difference between a player and a mack. The effects of a player are short-term, whereas the effects of a mack are long-term. As I mentioned earlier, all men have mackin' potential. They just have to tap into the mack within. When all men begin dating and becoming sexually active, they automatically become members of the proverbial T.M.A. (True Mack Association). Once you become a member of the T.M.A., you automatically receive 10 mackin' points, and the way you utilize your mackin' skills from that point on will determine whether your 10 mackin' points will be maintained or deducted. This is sort of like having a credit card. In some instances, when you are given a bank account, you automatically receive a credit card, and that card will have a certain limit on it. The way you use the card will determine if funds will be deducted or if more credit will be added. Once all the credit is relinquished, you are no longer a card member. The same goes with the T.M.A. Once all of your 10 mackin' points are deducted, you are no longer considered a true mack. (For example, if you cry in front of a woman, that's two (2) points deducted, and if you pay for sex, that's five (5) points deducted, etc.) There is nothing wrong with a man retiring his T.M.A. membership gracefully, and kickin' it with one female while living happily ever after. But if you claim to be in the mackin' game, you have to abide by the T.M.A. rules; otherwise, you are just talking the talk. And simply claiming the game doesn't make you a mack. You have to *live* the game. As I mentioned before, the information in this book can be applied to people who are trying to maintain normal, healthy, monogamous relationships, as well as aspiring macks. Since I was the world's first internationally known mackin' counselor,and game advisor, you can rest assured that my expertise is highly effective.

People with relationship problems have always come to those of us in the mackin' community for advice. Even boxing great Mike Tyson is said to have received marital advice from the legendary Iceberg Slim. One of the reasons I wanted to write this book is that many of my friends and associates (men and women), who sought my advice on problems they were having in relationships, told me that the advice I gave them changed their lives for the better. Some of these people had been to so-called professional counseling, only to receive no improving results. So, once the stereotypes, myths and misconceptions about macks are cleared up, you will understand that a true mack is indeed an asset to society.

"WE NEED TO INTERNALIZE THIS IDEA OF
EXCELLENCE. NOT MANY FOLKS SPEND A
LOT OF TIME TRYING TO BE EXCELLENT."

— BARACK OBAMA —

Chapter One

WHAT IS A TRUE MACK?

This chapter will help men look at female situations from a mack's point of view. I will point out how true macks deal with women from a *logical* standpoint instead of an *egotistical* standpoint. So, instead of being driven crazy, like the average brother, by a woman's many moods a true mack can calmly analyze the woman and deal with her accordingly, depending on her persona. But before you can learn about the woman's persona, you have to know and understand your own persona and objectives. Men are physical creatures and women are emotional creatures. Most men are only concerned with the superficial characteristics of women, and most women can detect this when they deal with men. Most women use logic and valid reasoning when dealing with men, and for the most part, women are clear on their objectives. This is why most women can outthink the average man. Once the woman has figured the man out, the game is over, because she now has him whipped, so to speak. The reason the game is over is because the woman is not intrigued anymore. It is human nature for people to mentally stimulate themselves by finding answers to the unknown. Take, for instance, putting the pieces of a jigsaw puzzle together. Once all the pieces of the puzzle are put together, you are not interested in that puzzle anymore, so it's on to the next game. One of the objectives of a true mack is to constantly add new pieces to that puzzle so that the woman will continue to be interested in his game. A true mack will always use logic in any situation. By using *logic,* a true mack can analyze a situation, then act accordingly. But a brother thinking with his ego will act on a situation without analyzing it and, therefore, play himself. For example, a woman may tell the square, average guy, "You are the sexiest man in the world." The square guy, thinking with his *ego,* will actually believe that he is the sexiest man in the world, and this allows the woman to then manipulate him. So, whenever the woman is trying to get over on the square, all she has to do is cater to his ego, and he will fall for anything, hook, line and sinker. Now, if a woman says to a mack, "You are the sexiest man in the world," a **mack,** using logic, will ask himself, "Why is she telling me this? Why is she trying to stroke my ego? What is she trying to gain?" This is how you figure out a woman's true *agenda.*

There are only three types of relationships, and this is one of the most important things a mack should know. People get into relationships for **emotional** gratification, *sexual* gratification and/or *financial* gratification. A woman may be in a relationship with a man whom she doesn't get along with emotionally, and his financial status may not be all that great, but he's real good in bed. That's a relationship based on *sexual* gratification. Or a man may be in a relationship with a woman who he isn't compatible with emotionally or sexually, but she helps him out with his car note, rent, etc. That's a relationship based *on financial* gratification. The job of a true mack is to figure out the woman's true agenda, because most women will not tell you overtly what their true agenda is. Some women pretend they want an emotional relationship with a man, when they're really just trying to get a few dollars out of him for next month's rent. This is why you use your *logic* instead of your *ego;* in using logic you can see past all the B.S. Now that you have a clear understanding of the types of relationships there are, it is time to analyze and understand what type of brother you are. There are generally two types of men: *squares* and *hustlers.* In the hustling category, there are three types: players, macks and pimps. There are also two types of players, the hustling player and the square player. A player's general objective is to have sexual encounters with as many women as possible. The hustling player will "play" until he realizes that it's time for him to graduate into mack status. He will then realize that he should at least receive some type of material gain as a result of his sexual encounters. But a square player has no desire for financial or material gain. He just wants to get as much sex as possible. If you are a man who is rolling in dough, there's nothing wrong with this. But if you're a brother who isn't ballin' like that, playing the field for recreational purposes is cool for a while, but at a certain point, you have to start playing to "come up." Since a player's' main objective is achieving sex from women, playin' is considered the simplest form of hustling. Pimpin' is considered the extreme form of hustling, because a true pimp's *only* objective is money, bottom line. The mack falls into that gray area between playin' and pimpin'. A mack is a brother who uses his verbal skills to attain his each and every goal, whether it's sex, money, love, employment, etc. A true mack can talk his way into and out of any situation. There's a saying in the hustling community that states, "Square players get played, pimps get paid, macks *persuade. So, basically, a true mack has we ability to get the paper, the power and the pussy.*

In the laymen society, there are generally four types of men. I refer to them as **the "4 P's"**:

Players (square players)

Professionals

Pushovers

Parolees

All four of these men have positive and negative attributes. Here is an analysis of the 4 P's.

Players

The good thing about players is they know what to say to women to stimulate them mentally. They also learn how to deal with a *number* of women fairly well. The hustlin' player has a high level of verbal game because he has to be very convincing to his women in order to come up on material items. But the square player doesn't really have any type of exceptional game. By using the slot machine technique (which I described before), he just happens to luck up on some ass every now and then. Although it is good for a player to continue rolling the dice until he makes a payoff, he should still use some form of strategy to help increase his chances of winning.

Many unseasoned, square players will lie, steal, cheat or do whatever it takes to get women into their bed. Almost every aspect of the square player's life revolves around him figuring out how to get new coochie. There's nothing wrong with wanting to get your freak on every now and then. But when it consumes every aspect of your life, and you have nothing to show for it, then you are playing yourself. Staying at the player level and not graduating to mack status is like staying in the twelfth grade for the rest of your life, and not graduating to college.

Professionals

The professional guy is usually a well educated brother. He usually comes from a stable family structure. He has been to the best schools, and he is used to all the finer things in life. These are the brothers who eventually become doctors, lawyers, accountants, executives and very astute businessmen. These brothers are disciplined, intelligent, financially stable and very goal-oriented. These are the positive aspects. On the flipside of the coin, these brothers often come off to women as being arrogant, pompous, snobby and stuck on themselves. The problem with these brothers is that they often seem to come off as narcissist, because they have a tendency to gloat about their accomplishments ("I got my B.A. from Harvard" or "I had to trade in my Benz today," etc.). These brothers are often critical of others and they sometimes look down on people that are not within their clique.

Pushovers

Pushovers are usually the hardworking, 9 to 5 men. These guys are usually easy going. They don't like to argue, and all they want is peace and harmony in their relationships. These are the men who know how to be sensitive with their women. These are the guys that will bring a woman flowers, open her car door for her, and call her at work throughout the day just to say "hi."

These guys usually try to avoid any conflict or confrontation with their women. These men generally want to settle down and just live one day at a time. On the negative side, these guys are usually looked upon by their women as having no backbone, and their women frequently walk all over them. These men generally grew up as mama's boys, and now they let their women call all the shots in the relationship. The pushover's woman will often test him by stepping to him in an aggressive manner, in the hope that he will eventually "be a man" and put her in check. Pushovers generally have no game, and they are known for tricking off their money on females in order to gain acceptance. Whenever a woman needs a bill paid, or a few dollars to hit the salon, all she has to do is call the pushover, and he will be there, at her command.

Parolees

These guys are usually the in-and-out-of-jail types of fellas. These men are also referred to as "thugs," "bad boys," "rough necks" and, erroneously, "gangsters." Many so-called gangsters would best be categorized as *bangers*. Gangsters and bangers are two different things. Real gangsters don't go in and out of jail, and they don't get caught up in little petty crimes. Real gangsters get their paper in a major way, whereas, most bangers tend to do dirt around their neighborhoods where they grew up. (A true gangster would fall into the category of the professional man.) The parolee is usually jobless, and if he does have a hustle, it's usually something like slangin' weed or serving rocks for a real gangsta. A lot of parolee guys tend to have a number of kids by a number of different women, and that too is one of his low-level hustles: The more baby-mamas he has, the more women that will be sending him care packages to the county jail the next time he gets locked up.

This is also the type of guy who sits in his woman's (or his mother's) house all day, smoking weed, playing video games, and thinking that he's pimpin'. But there is a big difference between *pimpin'* and *mooching.*

A lot of women are attracted to this type of guy because, with so many softhearted men out there on the dating scene, the parolee is the closest thing to a "real man" for these ladies. And women often get a sense of adventure from being with these so-called hard-core thugs. But the main reason women are attracted to this type of guy is because he's usually good in bed, and knows how to hit that ass right. Since this type of guy chooses not to make any significant social progress, he has lots of free time to master his bedroom skills, and he now knows that his sexual ability has become his trump card.

You should now have a basic understanding of the 4 P's. Of course, there are exceptions and there are also combination 4-P guys: There are some "professional-players" and some "pushover-parolees." But most men are either one extreme or the other, and my analogy is pretty accurate.

To many women, the ideal man is a combination of all the positive aspects of the 4 P's, and that is what a true mack is. A mack is smooth, and he knows how to properly deal with a number of women. Plus, he knows how to stimulate women mentally (like a player). A mack knows how to get his money, and he's very articulate and professional in his business dealings (like the professional). A mack knows how to be sensitive at the appropriate times. He knows how to do special little things for women every now and then. He knows how to handle problems without any major conflicts, and let the minor issues slide (like the pushover). And when it comes down to handling business in the bedroom with a female, a mack knows how to tap that ass like it is supposed to be tapped (like a parolee).

Although they hate to admit it, many women are intrigued by macks, because macks are a combination of all men. Macks are capable of covering all three of the relationship agendas because a true mack can satisfy a woman emotionally, financially and sexually.

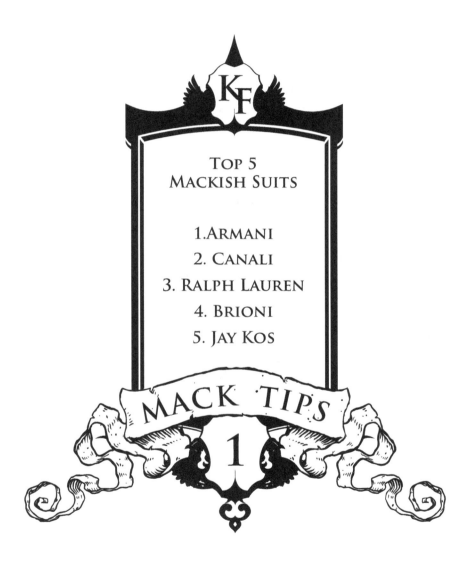

Top 5
Mackish Suits

1. Armani
2. Canali
3. Ralph Lauren
4. Brioni
5. Jay Kos

MACK TIPS

1

"WOMAN IS A MIRACLE OF
DIVINE CONTRADICTIONS."

— JULES MICHELET —

Chapter Two

THE FOUR TYPES OF FEMALES

To be successful in the art of mackin', an aspiring mack needs to know the type of women that he's dealing with. Understanding and figuring out a woman's many moods and characteristics has been a mystery to men since the beginning of time. That's why there are only a few true macks. Being able to deal with a woman's personality depends on many things, such as understanding her upbringing, knowing her geographical background, knowing the people she associates with, etc. Generally, there are four types of females, and within these categories there are many subcategories.

The four types of females are:

The Top-notch Female

The Middle-Class Girl

TheHoodrat

The Chickenhead

These women can also be referred to as the "4 H's":

The High-class Girl

The Homegirl

TheHoodrat

The Hoochie

Just like with the 4 P's, there are positive and negative aspects of the 4 H's. Let me break it down for you.

The High-class Girl (The Top-notch Female)

The high-class, top-notch female usually comes from a very stable home background, with both mother and father in the household. Since the father was usually present in this female's upbringing, she doesn't have to compensate later on in life by being hoochie in order to get that male attention. If the father was a hardworking, respectable man (which the topnotch female's father usually is), she knows what a real man is capable of. So, when it comes to choosing a mate later on in life, the high-class female would rather be by herself than settle for a nonproductive man.

Top-notch females are usually very well educated, focused and extremely driven when it comes to their careers. These women usually have good credit, and they are never delinquent when it comes to taking care of their bills. Most top-notch females maintain very nice, well-kept homes, and even though they may work long hours at the job, they at least make an effort to find time to keep their homes clean and presentable. Since these women are very confident with themselves, they don't have to dress hoochie or stank in order to get attention. They understand that a woman can be conservative and sexy at the same time.

Surprisingly, it is very hard for these females to find mates, because the average guy simply isn't on their level. High-class women are not impressed by the flossy, "I-got-money-and-a- Bentley" type of guy, because she has money of her own. In order to get with these women, you have to rely on straight verbal skills.

On the negative side, many of these females have a problem with playing the submissive role in their relationships. They are so used to being the boss and being in control of all other aspects of their lives, that they have a tendency to want to control the direction of their personal relationships as well. In many cases, they try to "out man the man." These women don't understand that in relationships there can't be two chiefs. Even though the male and female can be equal as far as their careers, ideas, etc., someone has to play the submissive role. And if that role is being played by the male, this will cause an imbalance in the relationship.

Top-notch women are also overly adamant about keeping their own identities. This is evident in why some professional top-notch women get married and keep their maiden names. (A lot of female doctors, lawyers, professionals, etc. have names like "Valerie Thomas-Smith" or "Lisa Johnson-Riley," etc.) Basically, when dealing with a top-notch woman, men have to really come correct.

The Homegirl (Middle-class Girl)

The middle-class girl usually has a girl-nextdoor type of quality. She is usually laid back and easy going. These girls usually come from a stable family background, and even if the father wasn't present in the home, she had a strongwilled mother who instilled good values in her. The homegirl usually grew up in a middle- to upper middle-class neighborhood. Unlike the top-notch female who, for the most part, only hangs out with other top-notch females, the middle-class girl has female friends and associates from all walks of life. She may have an occasional drink, or "hit the weed" every now and then, but she is generally not a heavy drug and alcohol user.

The middle-class girl usually has a regular 9 to 5 job that she is very content with. She may also have a decent, not-too-flashy automobile (on which she keeps up her payments). When dating, the middle-class girl doesn't make too many demands on her mate, and she is usually content with just staying home with her man and spending quality time. Her dress code is usually casual, yet tasteful, and she normally gets her clothes from the mall or other fashionable designer stores (not the swap meet). She usually keeps her feminine hygiene intact, and she tries to "hit the salon" on a weekly or biweekly basis.

Since most middle-class girls have such a down-to-earth attitude, men find them more approachable than other women. And because of this, these females tend to have relationships with a diverse group of men. On the negative side though, many middleclass girls have a tendency to be followers, and they often easily give in to peer pressure. These women usually don't possess the drive and leadership skills that are evident in the topnotch women; the middle-class girl likes to just roll with the in crowd.

Since the middle-class female has a strong family unit, her parents often act as her safety net. Because she can always fall back on her folks when times get rough, she usually doesn't have the incentive to take on any major responsibilities in life. This sometimes causes her to deal with certain issues in an immature way. But the middle-class girl is still considered the most desirable female to men.

The Hoodrat

When a female is considered a hoodrat, it is automatically assumed that this is something negative or derogatory. But the term hoodrat is not something that is necessarily negative, because hoodrats are just products of their environments. Basically, a hoodrat is a female that grew up (or still lives) in a low-income or impoverished neighborhood (the ghetto).

Most hoodrats grow up with no father in the home, and they often receive bad dating advice from all the different women in their lives. Since they grew up with no men in the household to set an example for them from a male perspective, hoodrats don't know how to deal with men when they get older. Many hoodrats tend to get into what I call "vicinity relationships." Since these women generally are not too worldly, their experiences are often limited to the events within their immediate neighborhoods. This, in turn, limits their dating options. Under these circumstances, these females are limited to only date the guys they grew up with, or the guys who live in the immediate vicinity. It's very common to meet a hoodrat who is in her mid- to late 20's, who has been dating the same guy since she was 16 or 17 years old. Even if she wanted to date another guy in her neighborhood, she can't because everybody knows each other. So in order to avoid the risk of conflict by dating one of her ex-boyfriend's "homies," she simply reconciles with the exboyfriend. Even if she does meet a guy from another neighborhood, he is not going to want to come around her and all of her ex-boyfriend's "homies." Basically, she gets stuck in these "vicinity relationships," because it is hard to break up with someone she is forced to see everyday, and who lives across the street or down the block from her.

There are two types of hoodrats:

The Round-the-way Girl
The Ghetto Queen

Although it is no one's choice to be born and raised in an impoverished neighborhood, the round-the-way girl has made a choice to at least try and work her way out of the hood, whereas the ghetto queen is totally content with her surroundings. The round-the-way girl is a hardworking sister who desperately wants to change her living condition. These women often have fulltime jobs, they go to school, and they sometimes have another part-time job to help make ends meet. Many round-the-way girls refuse to be pigeonholed into vicinity relationships. They would rather be by themselves and concentrate on bettering their living situations and careers than be forced, by circumstances, to date the "brothers from across the street."

Appearance-wise, the round-the-way girl often keeps her hair in a simple style such as braids, because with her work schedule and lack of disposable income, it's not easy for her to get her "do" done on a regular basis. For the most part, round-the-way girls are decent females who are trying to get themselves together. The ghetto queen, on the other hand, is somewhat of a hypocrite. The ghetto queen swears she is better than everybody else in the hood and looks down on other people, but she herself still lives in the projects.

Even though there are some ghetto queens that are attractive, well-kept young ladies, there are many that are only attractive to the guys in their neighborhoods. This type of ghetto queen is very popular amongst the guys around her way. The fellas have been jocking her since she was in junior high school, and this has caused her head to swell up tremendously. Since the ghetto queen has become so accustomed to praises and accolades from people in her hood, she has developed an innate fear of rejection and failure. She realizes that in the outside world, away from the hood, she has to compete with *real* women, and she would become just a grain of sand on a very big beach. Therefore, to avoid the risk of failure by venturing out into the world, she is content with staying in the ghetto so that the spotlight can remain on her, and she can stand out among the other hoodrats.

The Hoochie (The Chickenhead)

In the dating game, the chickenhead is on the bottom of the totem pole. **There are two types of chickenheads:**

The Low-budget Chickenhead

The Straight-up Hoochie Chickenhead

The only thing different about these two types of chickenheads is their appearance. Chickenheads generally come from broken homes where there are no father figures, and their mothers have dwelled in inferior living conditions as well. Instead of trying to better themselves, they continue to play the hoochie role, and then pass their chickenhead traits down to their daughters. This is why there are so many second and third generation chickenheads. Many mother-and-daughter chickenheads even hang out, get high and go to clubs together. To the mother chickenhead, she doesn't have a daughter, she has a kick it partner.

The chickenhead has no goals, no expectations or long-term outlook on life, and she is totally content with receiving her monthly county checks. Chickenheads normally have three to four kids by three to four different guys. Many dark-skinned chickenheads often try to have babies by light-skinned brothers because, in their feeble minds, they want their babies to come out with the proverbial "good hair."

Most chickenheads never move out of their parents' home, and if they do, they move into low-income or Section 8 housing. Even if a chickenhead uses Section 8 to move into a nice home, she will still keep her house nasty and filthy. In a chickenhead's home, you'll always find a bunch of guys just hanging out. And, in addition to her own children, she is always babysitting some other chickenhead's kids.

If you want peace and quiet, you won't find it in the home of a chickenhead, because she keeps the television up loud, the radio blasting, and a gang of kids running around screaming. Since most chickenheads don't have any type of real responsibilities, they can party and bullshit all day and all night as much as they please. Many chickenheads are excessive drinkers and marijuana users, and that is a double-edged sword, because weed makes them even more unmotivated and lazy. When the average chickenhead speaks, her voice is loud and raspy, due to cigarette smoking, heavy alcohol drinking and other drug use. In addition to having a loud and raspy voice, the chickenhead usually mispronounces her words and uses incorrect English. This is due primarily to lack of proper education and laziness, on her part, to not want to better her verbal skills.

Even if a chickenhead is on Section 8, she still has to pay at least some of the utility bills, and for her, even that is a struggle. She's constantly getting her phone disconnected, and when she does get it turned back on, she has it in one of her kid's name. The only bill that a chickenhead will faithfully pay on time is the cable bill. A chickenhead can tell you about every video that's playing on B.E.T., every guest on the latest daytime talk show, and what's happening on the "stories."

When her phone is not disconnected, she calls up her other chickenhead friends all day and gossips about all the productive people in society. She lets her children walk around dirty, with Kool-Aid stains on their clothes and unruly hairstyles. One good thing to say about some chickenheads is that, because of their food stamps and WIC vouchers, they do keep a house full of food. Appearancewise, the low-budget chickenhead and the straight-up hoochie chickenhead go from one extreme to the other. The *hoochie* tries too much and the *low-budget* female doesn't try hard enough. The lowbudget female will walk around with a weave that doesn't match her real hair, her shoes will be beat up and run over, and her feet will be dry and ashy. Since most "low-budget" females don't have cars, the bottom of their ankles usually have scab marks on them as a result of walking around in bad shoes. When the low-budget female does leave the house, she normally goes to her four favorite places: the county building, the swap meet, the market and the liquor store (to get her liquor and blunts).

My definition of a hoochie is a woman who overly accentuates herself. Many women go through somewhat of a hoochie stage between the ages of 17 and 21. When a female reaches the age of 17 or 18, her body is starting to fully develop. At this point, she has ass and titties that weren't there before. And with these new and developed body parts, there also comes new attention from guys that wasn't there before either. Now that she sees men are sweating her because of her new physical appearance, she becomes very confident about her body, and she wants to accentuate her most intriguing "assets." Most females grow out of the "flaunting-my body" stage in a couple of years, because they realize that all attention is not good attention. They also realize that by age 21 they haven't had a real, meaningful relationship that was not based strictly on their physical attributes alone, so now they concentrate on getting their minds right.

The chickenhead hoochie, on the other hand, stopped focusing on her mind altogether and continued to focus primarily on her physical appearance. Since the average hoochie is basically broke, she tries to over compensate by at least trying to look successful. She does this by wearing loud, flashy clothes; long, elaborate acrylic fingernails; and lots of gaudy jewelry. She doesn't realize that most financially successful people are generally conservative in their physical appearance, and they have no need to floss and front. But the hoochie is satisfied with *looking* like a ghetto celebrity.

Hoochies also like to wear big, extravagant hairstyles with many different shapes and colors. (Some hoochies even put shiny glitter on their hair and faces.) Hoochies oftentimes wear their makeup in weird patterns, and they sometimes have up to 10 or 12 earrings in each ear. Many hoochies wear clothes that are two sizes too small, and they often wear outfits that are obviously inappropriate for certain occasions. It's not surprising to see a hoochie go into a funeral wearing a red leather mini-skirt, or going to a gospel concert wearing an orange catsuit.

One thing about a hoochie is that she can be living in squalor, but she is going to make sure that her hair and nails are done by the weekend. Many men have to be very careful when it comes to dealing with chickenheads. Sometimes these women will try to pass themselves off as plain hoodrats or disguise themselves as middle-class girls. (It's almost impossible for a chickenhead to pass herself off as a topnotch.) A true mack doesn't deal with chickenheads on a regular basis. If he does, it is just for recreational purposes, or to have as a platonic friend.

I've compiled a list of ways you can tell if a woman is a chickenhead when you meet her. When you first meet a woman, normally, she tries to present herself in the most interesting way possible. But it's the nonverbal communication that you should focus on. It's really the little things that say a lot about a person.

Here is a list of the **20 ways to tell if a woman may be a chickenhead (low-budget or hoochie):**

1. If she smacks her gum.
2. If she has chipped fingernail polish.
3. If her weave doesn't match her real hair.
4. If her lips are purple from smoking weed.
5. If she's trying to show off her navel ring and she has a gang of stretch marks.
6. If she's at the mall in house shoes and hair rollers.
7. If she's loud and flamboyant.
8. If she has gold teeth.
9. If she has nappy, sweaty braids.
10. If she has on lipstick with eyeliner pencil around her lips.
11. If she is wearing a skirt and you can see panty lines and cellulite through the skirt.
12. If she has cocoa butter on her neck and forehead because she burned herself trying to do her own hair.
13. If she and her friends are wearing matching outfits from the swap meet.
14. If she's eight months pregnant and still going to the club.
15. If she has teeth missing.

16. If she has acrylics on her *toenails.*

17. If she's wearing an evening dress with tennis shoes.

18. If she still has the price tag on her outfit, so that she can take it back to the store when she's through wearing it.

19. If her stomach is too big to be exposed, ... and it's exposed.

20. If she's impressed with guys who have nice rims on their cars.

Now, if you have encountered a woman with some of these characteristics, but you are still not sure if she is a chickenhead or not, don't worry. All you have to do is go into a woman's home and look at her surroundings. This will **really** help validate what type of woman she is. Most chickenheads keep their homes filthy and deplorable.

But when company is expected, she may try and tidy up a bit. In some cases, in order to keep up the facade of appearing normal, some chickenheads even have the nerve to have a family pet in the home. If they do have a pet, such as a cat or a dog, usually the poor animal is walking around the house starving, looking more like a *hostage* than anything else. No matter what a woman projects to you, there are certain clues to look for when you are in her home. These clues will give you a much better understanding of her and her personality

So here is a list of **10 ways to tell if you are in the home of a chickenhead:**

1). If her home has that fried chicken and urine smell.
2). If there are four or more kids running around.
3). If all the food in the kitchen consists of milk, cheese and cereal products.
4). If she has on an ankle bracelet because she's on house arrest.
5). If you go to use her telephone and the receiver smells like "stank breath."
6). If her mother tries to send you to the store for "beer."
7). If she has a pet dog and you can see its rib cage.
8). If her phone is ringing nonstop.
9). If she washes her panties in the bathroom sink.
10).If her grandmother just got back in/town from All Star Weekend

(I know it may seem that I'm trying to make jokes, but I have actually witnessed, and experienced, everything that was just mentioned.)

One of the most interesting things about chickenheads is that, surprisingly, they don't have too much trouble finding male companionship. Since men figure that they can get with these women with little, if any, effort, chickenheads are considered easy access.

Even though I come off hard on these women, in all fairness, most chickenheads aren't bad people. They just need self-confidence and self-motivation to get up and do better for themselves.

Now that you have a general understanding of the four types of females that are on the dating scene, you need to become familiar with some of the subcategories of women. You also need to know how to deal with these women correctly. Sometimes the way a mack kicks his game depends on the geographical background of the woman he's mackin' to.

Because I have lived in many different cities across the country, I've learned that a mack's game has to be flexible and able to culturally adapt. (Of course, there are many exceptions, but there are some basic things that you should know that will, at least, get you in the right frame of mind when dealing with women in different parts of the country.)

For instance, the women in the South usually live plain, simple lives. Their towns are very close knit, so they've been knowing the same people and seeing the same things most of their lives. (This is especially so for females who live in rural parts of the South.) So when you spit game at these Southern girls, you have to be imaginative and colorful with your words. You have to come off as being exciting and intriguing. A lot of Southern rural females love men from other cities because they are a break from the norm. Not too many things out of the ordinary happen in these small, rural Southern towns, so the females are easily captivated by seemingly fast paced men from major cities.

Now, West Coast women are totally different. A typical woman from a city like Los Angeles is not easily impressed by glitz and glamour (unless she's a chickenhead), because L.A. is the floss capital of the world. In a town where celebrities are seen on the regular, and frontin 'n flossin is the norm, a mack will stand out more if he uses the laid-back-and-honest approach.

When dealing with West Coast women, an aspiring mack should never brag about his material possessions or the people he knows. That routine is played out, and these women will look at you as being a buster or a square. (I will go into detail about making your approach in later chapters.) When dealing with a West Coast female who has the Hollywood mentality, consider her open game for putting your "smooth player" mack down. Since these females aren't living in reality anyway, any type of relationship that does stem from the two of you will most likely be short-term, so you might as well mack up on some ass.

When dealing with the Hollywood type of female, you should limit the information you give about yourself and let your personal background remain a mystery. (This is done strictly for the purpose of intrigue.) And since Hollywood is a place where people are considered very narcissistic, encourage the Hollywood female to talk about her favorite subject, herself. Once you get her in a comfort zone, you then step up your mackin', and go in for the kill, so to speak.

With women from Eastern cities (such as Chicago, Detroit, New York, etc.), you have to come at them with a little more sternness and aggressiveness. A lot of men are intimidated by women from Eastern cities, because a lot of these women have a no-nonsense, and sometimes rigid, disposition. You must understand that in a city like Detroit or New York, there's a fast-paced, hustle-and-bustle mentality in the air. Plus, it's too cold to bullshit, so these women want you to come correct immediately, or don't come at all. A real mack doesn't let these women intimidate him, and he steps to them with the same rigor and firmness that *they* exude. These women can smell weakness from a mile away, so you have to step to them with total confidence and authority. Although I have given you a generalized view of all the types of women that are out in the dating market place, there are some other personality traits and dysfunctions that you should become familiar with. Most of these dysfunctions in women are universal, and can be found in any one of the 4 P's. One of the rules of mackin' is to avoid as many problems as possible. Your main objective is to screen as many women as possible to see which ones are the most receptive to your game. When dealing with a female who has issues, you have to be extremely cautious. You could end up wasting valuable mackin' time on a situation that's simply not going to amount to anything, no matter how tight your game is. Mackin' to a dysfunctional female, or a woman that you are simply not compatible with, is like digging for a diamond in a sandbox. You could have the best, most high-tech digging equipment in the world, but you are simply not going to find a diamond in certain vicinities.

Here is a list of the **top five dysfunctional women to watch out for:**

1).The Drama Queen
2).The Rebound Chick
3).The Sanctified, Shy Girl
4).Madam Maybelline
5).The Psycho Wench

Now, with some of these women you may just well have a beneficial relationship, but from my own experiences and analysis, I suggest you do so with extreme caution. Here is a rundown of these females:

The Drama Queen
This female is not satisfied unless there is some type of crisis happening in her life. She's the type of person who blows everything out of proportion, and she goes to emotional extremes. One minute she's crying and the next minute she's raving mad. She does this because, in reality, her life is relatively boring, and she feels that she has to create a more extravagant, alternative life in her mind. In essence, she creates so much drama because she simply has nothing better

to do. Drama queens are overly paranoid and delusional, and they often falsely accuse people of conspiring against them. You'll often hear drama queens say things like, "My whole family is against me" or "The people at my job are out to destroy me." Oftentimes, we just want to grab the drama queen and say, "Look, it ain't that serious!"

This woman will get overly emotional about every little thing, and it doesn't take much to set her off. All she needs is a little "ammo," and her "drama guns" will start shooting. **Here are some examples of drama queen symptoms:** *If she goes off on the McDonald's worker for not putting cheese on her Big Mac, or for not putting extra salt on her fries.

*If she files sexual harassment charges against a co-worker because he gave her an innocent compliment.

*If you just met her for the first time at a club or a social function, and she gets mad when she sees you talking to another woman.

*If you show up five minutes late for a date and she says something like, "Oh, you're late. Now you've ruined the evening! Now we can't go anywhere!"

If any of these characteristics sound familiar, more than likely you are dealing with a straight up drama queen, and I suggest you tighten up your game.

The Rebound Chick

The rebound chick is a female who is fresh out of a bad relationship or who is currently on shaky terms with her significant other. If you meet a female who says that she just "broke up with her man a week ago," or that she and her man are on "bad terms right now," she wants to do one of two things:

* get an ego boost
* or get revenge.

This type of female wants to immediately go out and meet new men so that they can hopefully cater to her ego. Because of her failed relationship, at this point she is vulnerable and she has a lot of self-doubt. All she wants is a brother to, at least, give her the *impression* that she is significant, sexy, interesting or just plain **wanted.** But a female who is just on bad terms with her mate normally has a different agenda. Oftentimes, she wants to get a conscious or subconscious form of revenge on her mate by hurting him the way he has hurt her. By meeting and hooking up with other guys, she feels that she is getting some form of payback on her mate. If you meet a woman like this, you have to realize that a meaningful, long-term relationship with her is normally out of the question, and the only relationship you could possibly have with her is a sexual one, which is not so bad. But there's a catch. If you do decide that you want to have a sexual encounter with a rebound chick, the encounter will have to take place as soon as possible. In most cases, you have a three-day period in which to have sexual relations with a rebound chick. (That's right ... you have 72 hours to get the coochie.) These females don't stay mad at their mates for too long, and it's inevitable that they are going to try to reconcile their differences. This usually happens within a two- to three-day period (especially if she's living with her man). So, as a mack, you have to step up your game, and get that ass before she gets back with her man. (I will explain how to actually get the ass in Chapter 6.) Now, I know that these tactics may sound crude and deceptively manipulative, but the rebound chick is being somewhat manipulative herself. She gives the impression that she is interested in these men so that they can give her attention, and cater to and help build up her selfesteem. And when they do, she kicks them to the curb and goes back to her mate. As the saying goes, game recognize game, and as a mack, always stay on top of your game.

The Sanctified, Shy Girl

In all fairness, there is nothing wrong with a female being a little shy, but when she is overly shy, that should signal a caution light. Shyness can have positive and negative implications. Some seemingly shy women are simply *reserved.* Some of these females keep their emotions so pinned up inside, when they do have a vehicle, such as sex, to release all that emotional energy, they seem to get buck wild. It's an open secret in the mackin' community that shy girls are the freakiest females, which is not a bad thing. The ideal woman for most men is the closet freak. But some of these so-called shy girls have many skeletons in their closets, and they can get a little *too* freaky with too many people. These women act shy because they've become insecure and fearful that if they reveal too much about themselves, others will learn of their tainted past.

There may be a number of contributing factors to the overly shy girl's behavior. She may have had a threesome in high school; she could have been a stripper in college; she could have done a porno movie because she was in a financial bind; or she could have gotten drunk and had sex with a goat. Who knows? The point is that many of these women have done so much freaking in their past, that they now they feel they need some type of *spiritual cleansing,* and they now start overemphasizing the need to go to church. There's nothing wrong with going to church or having some type of spiritual involvement. But if you meet an extremely attractive woman who is playing the sanctified, miss-goodie-two-shoes role a little bit too well, keep an eye on her. Sure, there are many good women out there, but when something seems a little too good to be true, you should be cautious. The sanctified, shy girl might have had a past so stank that she now needs divine intervention. She may be the kind of girl that has screwed half the brothers in the NBA, and now she claims she's "saved." She has basically freaked every brother in her social circle, and since there is no one else left to freak (and since all her freaking partners have kicked her to the curb), she now turns to the church. In many cases, if you give one of these so-called sanctified girls a sip of Long Island Iced Tea, she'll be back to her old hoochie ways. People can't put up "fronts" for too long, and the truth will always make itself known. Some of these shy, sanctified women only get saved when it's convenient for them. On Saturday night they're at the club drunk, and backing that ass up. And on Sunday morning they're in church asking the reverend to rebuke the "stank demons" from them. So beware of the so-called shy girl, because she may be "stanktified."

Madam Maybelline

Madam Maybelline is the type of female who wears entirely too much makeup. Instead of using makeup to simply highlight or accentuate her natural features, Madam Maybelline paints on an entirely *new face*. In most cases, when you see this type of female without her makeup on, she looks like a totally different person. Anyone can get that glamorous, feminine look if they plaster on a ton of makeup (take crossdressing singer "RuPaul," for example).

Madam Maybelline's heavily made up look is somewhat deceptive, because she is presenting a *caricature* of who she really is. When women go out with an excessive amount of makeup on, the message they send out is, "I'm so insecure about my facial features that I have to hide behind all of these cosmetics."

Now, if a woman is an entertainer or if she is appearing in front of a camera, wearing a certain amount of makeup is justified. But if a female is putting on a gang of makeup just to go to the mall, she may have issues. This type of female may have problems with insecurity, and I advise all aspiring macks to beware.

The Psycho Wench

Don't be fooled by the so-called psycho wench. In most cases, this type of female just likes to play crazy. The "psycho wench" normally has had a trail of failed relationships that she probably tried to reconcile in positive ways. Since that didn't work, she now has a new way of dealing with men in relationships. If a man does something that *she* considers deceptive or untrustworthy, her reaction is to play psycho and scare the man into submission. She figures that if she acts this way men will think, "I'd better not do anything wrong to this woman, because there's no telling what this woman will do to me."

This type of female is extremely insecure, and her behavior is very compulsive. When dealing with a man, she will act overly jealous; she will page his beeper 20 times in a row;

she will call his home leaving threatening messages on his answering machine; she will snoop through his belongings; she will hide out in the bushes in front of his house; she will try to physically fight him in public; and she will curse out his mama. She will basically act like a total idiot just to prove that "she ain't to be fucked with."

The old school pimps categorized this behavior as "playing the nut roll." That's exactly what she's doing, playing the roll of a nut. It is all an act. When a female pulls her little "psycho routine" on a real mack, he is neither intimidated nor fazed by it. You have to put these women in check, and check 'em hard. You let them know that they can rant and rave ail they want, but a mack is still running things. Once she sees that you are not intimidated by her antics, she will regroup and come at you like she has some sense.

Subconsciously, these women want a man to stand up and put them in check for a change. The psycho roll is really just a test. (Many hookers do this to qualify a pimp. More on that in the next chapter.) For the most part, the psycho wench routine that some women pull is harmless. But be warned: There are some psycho wenches out there that *will* stab your ass, so be careful. A true-to-form psycho wench won't do all that ranting and raving and screaming and hollering. She is calm and emotionless. This is the type of female that will catch you when you are vulnerable. She will wait until you go to sleep, or until you are taking a shower, then she will come in the room with a boiling hot bowl of Cream of Wheat and throw it on you, or something of that nature. So realize that there are some females out there that you don't want to cross.

Now you have a basic understanding of some of the sisters that are out there on the dating scene. Remember, do not be manipulated or misled by what some of these women *tell* you about themselves, because as I mentioned earlier, many people try to present themselves as being better than what they really are. As a mack, you have to listen with your eyes. You have to read body language and other nonverbal communication in order to get a better understanding of the women you deal with.

As I also mentioned before, none of the women in this chapter are universally good or bad. One man's "bed wench" may be another man's queen. There are positive and negative traits to all of these women (even the chickenheads), but a true mack wants to stick with the high-class woman or the "homegirl" (and, in some cases, the round-the-way hoodrat) and put the other women in the platonic zone. (More on the platonic zone in later chapters.)

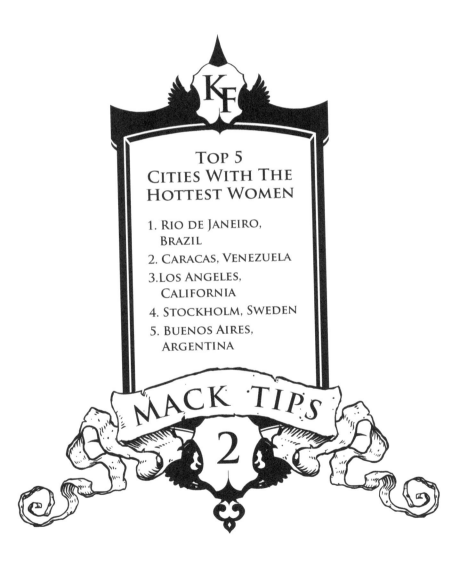

TOP 5 CITIES WITH THE HOTTEST WOMEN

1. RIO DE JANEIRO, BRAZIL
2. CARACAS, VENEZUELA
3. LOS ANGELES, CALIFORNIA
4. STOCKHOLM, SWEDEN
5. BUENOS AIRES, ARGENTINA

MACK TIPS

2

"DISAPPOINTINGLY ENOUGH,
WHEN ONE LEARNS TO CONTROL EIGHT
OR NINE OR TEN WOMEN; THEN ALL THE
LUSTER, ALL THE GLORY IS GONE."

— ICEBERG SLIM —

Chapter Three

THE PIMP MENTALITY

The purpose of writing this chapter about The pimp mentality is not to influence the reader to actually become a pimp (so don't run out and put a down payment on a fur coat and a Cadillac). What I *do* want to get across to you is a real understanding of the pimp game and what a pimp goes through. Pimping is the extreme form of mackin', and one has to admit that it takes some serious game for a brother to have a stable of women breakin' him off paper on the regular. So in this chapter I want you, the reader, to take some of the rules and knowledge of the pimp game and apply it to some of your not-so extreme relationships.

First of all, I need to clear up some of the stereotypes and misconceptions about the pimp game. Society has been subjected to the *Hollywood* perception of the pimp game. This is partly due to the fact that the actual pimping community is very close-knit and secretive.

Since society doesn't often receive information from actual pimpin' participants, people often rush to judgment and come to their own conclusions. The image of the pimp that most people are familiar with is the Superfly-Dolimite looking brother, wearing outrageously colorful costumes, while driving around in an orange Cadillac, slapping his hoes. Sure, there are pimps that are synonymous with this image, but they are a very small fraction of the pimpin' community.

A legendary Los Angeles pimp known as Rosebudd once told me that it's easy to turn out new girls, because they don't know how to look out and stay away from a *real* pimp. Since these girls are so busy looking out for "Huggy Bear," when a real pimp does roll up on them, it's too late.

Here are the four biggest misconceptions about pimps:

1). Pimps force helpless women into a life of prostitution
Society seems to think that all pimps are low-life scumbags, who hang around bus stations, turning out teenage runaways. People would like to think that all pimps *prey* on women, but in most cases, hoes *choose* pimps. There are many contributing factors that make women want

to become whores and, in most cases, these females are whores long before the pimp gets to them. If you look at the way these middle school and high school girls dress and carry on in different cities across the country, you can see the ones that are potential whores. This has more to do with their upbringing than the intervention of the pimp. In many cases, it's the girl's family that "turns her out," so to speak. The pimp comes along after the fact, to at least give her some guidance in her unfortunate profession. Every woman has a need for companionship, and the prostitute is not exempt. Tricks and squares don't want the prostitute for anything beyond receiving their own sexual gratification. So the only man that is compatible with the whore is the pimp. The pimp is there for emotional support and financial guidance. The pimp is her guiding light, her father figure, her manager and many other things. This is why most hoes *choose* pimps: He is the only male that she considers a real man. Sure, there are many cases where pimps turn out underage girls, but this is an exception, not the norm.

2). Pimps are oversexed perverts who are constantly having orgies with their whores
Many misguided young men want to get in the pimp game

because they think that it is a sexual free-for-all. Nothing can be further from the truth. People seem to believe that a pimp performs some type of sexually outrageous act on women in order to turn them out or to get them in his stable. But pimpin' is not a *sexual* game. It's a **mental** game. The pimp understands that one must control the woman's mind before he can control her body or her finances. A good pimp rarely, if ever, has sexual relations with his girls. A pimp understands that there are tricks and Johns that will freak his whores into a frenzy, and have them cumming for days.

So there's nothing that a pimp can do sexually that hasn't been done to his girls before. The pimp is the antithesis to the trick. The pimp is the only man that is not hounding the prostitute for sex. When a trick steps to a prostitute, he is trying to pay for sex. When a square steps to a prostitute, he is trying to con her out of free sex. But the pimp will step to her on another level. He is the only man who refuses her sexual favors, and this is one of the things that keep the prostitute intrigued with him. If a pimp *does* decide to have sex with one of his girls, he uses it as a form of reward to her. He might do this because she has reached a monetary quota that he has set for her. Some pimps just straight up charge hoes a freaking fee before they engage in any sexual act with them. Pimps mainly do this for psychological purposes. By having casual sex with his hoes and not charging them, the pimp runs the risk of having his hoes lose respect for him, because now he's acting like a trick and a square. One of the main rules of pimpin' is to not hound your hoes for sex, because if you do, you will lose them in a heartbeat.

3). Pimps keep their hoes held hostage and they "strong arm" money from them

For years, society has been stumped on why hoes stay with their pimps. People would like to think that a pimp has to keep his women chained up in the house so they can't leave, but that too is anti-pimp propaganda. The main reason a woman stays with a pimp is because the pimp gets the woman to *invest* in him. When a whore steps to a pimp, she normally has to have some type of choosing money to give to him. (I like to refer to this as "making a deposit.") Again, this is done for psychological purposes. The pimp understands that the more money a woman invests, the least likely she is to walk away from her investment. (This is why it is important for the women to initially make a deposit.)

This is the same as Wall Street investing. If an investor plays the stock market and buys 20,000 shares of a company, even if the company goes through financial ups and downs, the investor is not going to immediately walk away from his investment. He is going to ride it out to see if it gets better, and hopefully cash in on his investment.

The same thing goes with a whore investing in a pimp. The pimp presents the prospect of her having a better living situation if she joins his stable. On the strength of his prospects and potential, the whore immediately puts down a deposit with the particular pimp. If she has invested 30 or 40 thousand dollars of her "trap money" into a pimp, she is going to be reluctant about walking away from him, regardless of any problems or differences they may have.

A pimp doesn't physically have to keep his hoes on lock down, because he has them mentally locked. This is the same reason square women stay in bad relationships with square men. These women are also reluctant to leave their relationships because they have invested so much *time* and *energy* to make it work. So the square girl is no different than the call girl in regards to staying in so-called dysfunctional relationships. (And square girls are just as inclined to invest their money in these relationships as well.) Another rule of the pimp game is, "If she likes you, she'll pay you."

4). Pimps are weasel-like characters who dress in loud, tasteless clothing

Sure, there are some pimps that are overly flashy, but in many cases, pimps are conservative in their attire and demeanor. A smart pimp plays the low key role (unless he is out campaigning for new girls) and doesn't try to draw too much negative attention to himself or his stable. As the legendary Chicago pimp Bilbo Gholson stated in his book, The Pimp's Bible, a real pimp shouldn't "play the game and escape the name." He also shouldn't drive around in a pink, convertible Cadillac wearing a big ass purple hat tilted to the side, with an eight-track tape player bumping the theme from Shaft.

A real pimp doesn't have to scream out (verbally or nonverbally), "I'm a pimp!" His pimpin' should show naturally. Hollywood is to blame, in part, for the Huggy Bear image of the pimp game. Unfortunately, there are some pimps who cater to that Hollywood image, and this is the image that society accepts for all pimps. HBO ran a special on its cable network called "Pimps Up, Hoes Down," and many pimps I know had a lot of harsh criticism for the documentary. These pimps felt that many of the participants were cartoon-like and buffoonish, and that they only represented a very minute sector of the pimp world. There are many other misconceptions about the pimp game, but the ones that I just stated are the most common. What is important for people to know is that pimping is a lifestyle and a *profession*. And, in any profession, there are going to be positive individuals and negative individuals, but the negative individuals shouldn't represent the whole conglomerate.

Another reason that society comes to negative conclusions about the pimp game is because of a lack of knowledge and understanding about the game. Pimping is considered the oldest game, but as rapper/actor Ice-T once stated, pimping is the *only* game.

The prerequisite for pimping is *capitalism*. In a system of capitalism, a person has to capitalize off the work of others. The very definition of capitalize means "to profit from" or "to exploit." Society often accuses pimps of exploiting women, but if a person puts in 40 hours a week at a regular job, making their boss richer and richer, technically, they are also being exploited to a certain degree.

In any employment situation, you are going to be a pimp or you are going to be a ho, and the terms "pimp" and "ho" are just euphemisms for the terms "boss" and "employee." But the term pimping, in relation to prostitution, didn't come into play until after slavery.

When the slaves were freed in the South, many of these Black men and women moved north to reconstruct their lives and to find employment. When the White men in these northern cities came into contact with these newly-migrated Black women, they became intrigued with their natural sexuality. So these White men began to pursue sexual exploits with these black women. Many of these women engaged in sexual exploits with these men because they felt they still had to be somewhat legally subservient to Whites. But the Black men reminded these sisters that they were not on the plantation anymore, and that they didn't have to engage in sex because "massah said so." Basically, these Black men told these women to have the White men break them off some money before they do anything with them. The Black men took their cut of the money, and this is how pimping began in the Black community.

Even then, people were amazed by pimps. These ex-slaves started off with visibly nothing, and ended up with just as much as, if not more than, many well-off Whites at that time. Today, pimpin' is considered a victimless crime, because all three benefactors—the pimp, the ho and the trick—are willing participants in this endeavor. In no way am I trying to glorify the pimp/prostitution lifestyle, because this isn't a glamorous game.

In a very indirect way, pimps capitalize off the misfortunes of others. But this is no different from, say, the medical profession. Doctors benefit from the illnesses and injuries of others. This isn't to say that doctors and surgeons just sit around in emergency rooms hoping for people to get shot and stabbed. But if a person does have the misfortune of sustaining an injury, they are entitled to the best medical assistance possible, and the doctor will provide that. If a woman has the misfortune of becoming a prostitute, the pimp is there to assist her through her chosen career path.

As I stated earlier, most prostitutes are already turned out when they do decide to choose a pimp. There are dozens of reasons that contribute to women becoming prostitutes. It could be something as extreme as the female having been molested as a child, or something as simple as her not having a father figure while growing up and now she's desperately seeking any kind of male attention. Or it could be that the woman is in a financial bind, and she thinks that prostitution is her last resort.

There are generally four types of prostitutes,
and they are:

1).The Call Girl

2).The Streetwalker

3).The Part-time Prostitute

4).The Stank Ho

Here is a brief rundown of all four:

The Call Girl

The call girl is considered the high-class prostitute. This woman normally operates through some type of escort or outcall agency that is normally set up by highly organized pimps. She usually caters to an upscale clientele, and her fee could start at $500 to $1000 an hour.

In addition to her upfront fee, she usually requires tips for any additional services. The call girl carries herself in a very professional manner, and it is usually hard to distinguish her from a top-notch square. This is why many ballers, shot callers, professional athletes and entertainers associate themselves with these two types of women. In many cases, if a man is financially stable, he wants a financially stable square or a financially stable ho. Nothing in between. Call girls are financially stable: They dress in the highest fashions and drive the fanciest cars. The call girl has decided that, if she is going to be a ho, she is going to be the best ho.

The Streetwalker

These are the women that flip in and out of cars while

working the track. As King Bilbo stated in his book, many of these women are unclean and a lot of them carry diseases. In many cases, if a streetwalker doesn't have a pimp, she's usually trying to support a drug habit. All she wants to do is trick up enough money for her "hit" and hotel fare. A chili pimp (a pimp with one whore) will go broke trying to work a streetwalker. In order for a pimp to make any money off of this type of prostitute, he would have to have a whole stable of streetwalkers working different tracks at different times.

The Part-time Prostitute (The Weekend Warrior)

The part-time prostitute is a woman who tries to live a double life. This type of woman has a square job in the daytime, and she works for an escort agency, after-hours joint, or a strip club at night. Many of these women live a totally square life during the week, and on weekends they travel out of town to cities like Las Vegas or Atlantic City and work the tracks there.

These women are commonly referred to by law enforcement agents as "weekend warriors." These women are easy to turn out because they are basically halfway there. So all a pimp has to do is talk some common sense into them. He questions them on why they would work in a strip club, doing $10 table dances and performing flips and acrobatics for $1 tips, when they could be making $500 an hour.

Women from different square professions moonlight as weekend warriors, but the most common ones are schoolteachers. The reason for this may be that many female educators are so underpaid in their professions, they feel that they have to turn tricks on the side to make ends meet. Many women who work in strip clubs are also considered part-time prostitutes. Although many strippers claim that they do not turn tricks, and that they are not prostitutes, I can assure you that the majority of them will turn a trick every now and then, if the price is right.

The Stank Ho

This female is considered the lowest form of hooker. The stank ho almost doesn't deserve to be in the category of prostitution, because if she does decide to receive material gains from her sexual exploits, it's usually menial items such as weed, a trip to the nail shop, crack or food. The stank ho basically likes to have sex for recreation. She is considered the neighborhood freak. She is a loose, malicious woman who lacks sexual discipline. Many stank hoes consider themselves square, and they have a lot of criticism for women who openly sell sex.

If a normal prostitute is going to have numerous sex partners, at least she has enough sense to get paid. But the stank ho is content with fucking guys for Happy Meals.

Knowing and understanding these four types of prostitutes has a lot to do with the way a pimp deals with them. In order to be a good pimp, you have to know how these women think and what motivates them. The way a pimp handles his business depends on the type of pimp he is.

"King Bilbo" states in his book that there are 52 versions of the pimp, but I believe **most pimps generally fall into five basic categories.** They are:

The Gorilla Pimp
The Sweet Mackin' Pimp
The Rigid Pimp
The Professional Pimp
The Overly Flashy Pimp

Here is a rundown of all five types of pimps:

The Gorilla Pimp

The gorilla pimp is usually a big, huge bully type or a short, feisty brother with a little man's complex. This type of pimp loves beating on his hoes. Overtly, he claims this is necessary to keep his hoes in check but, in reality, he does this because it gives him a sense of power. His game isn't exceptionally tight, and "kicking off in a bitch's ass" is his trump card. He pimps off of fear, not respect.

The Sweet Mackin' Pimp

This is a smooth, suave, sweet-talking type of pimp. His verbal skills are almost hypnotic to women, and it is his charisma that gets him over. He tells his hoes everything they want to hear. This type of pimp makes all his hoes feel special, and he always knows the right thing to say at the right time. The sweet mackin' pimp is real good at turning girls out, because younger females are very receptive to his game.

The Rigid Pimp

The rigid pimp is the no-nonsense type of pimp. He usually

has strict rules and guidelines that his girls must abide by, and he is very uncompromising. He rarely, if ever, gets physical or violent with his girls. But if he does have to use violent tactics to take disciplinary actions on one of his girls, he will have his "bottom bitch" administer the actual physical act on the said subject. The rigid pimp is adamant about his girls meeting their quotas and he will accept no excuses. If he has his women going through an agency, and business there is slow, he won't hesitate to tell his girls to "take off your *low heels,* and put on your *ho heels,*" and he'll put them right on the track.

The Professional Pimp

This type of pimp runs his stable as if it were a legitimate business. He normally has some type of escort agency set up, and he really screens the women that choose him. In some cases, this type of pimp even makes his new recruits fill out an actual job application to keep on file. This pimp is very conservative, and if any problems arise concerning his females, he handles them with diplomacy and professionalism.

The Overly Flashy Pimp

This is the pimp that all other pimps are stereotyped after. He drives around in overaccessorized cars and wears loud clothes, with huge hats that have feathers in them. And, in most cases, his hoes are just as obnoxious and tacky as he is. He can only pimp on low-budget, ghetto chicks because they are the only women who are impressed with his antics.

Rosebudd once told me that the reason Hollywood created the image of the pimp wearing blouse-like shirts, skin-tight pants, highheeled shoes, loud, flamboyant colors and other overly exaggerated costumes is because White men have always wanted to portray the pimp as some type of homosexual figure. The fact that these Black men had the ability to control the minds of numerous women, strictly by using their verbal skills, made White men feel like they had to de-emasculate the image of the pimp. So, in the 70's, Hollywood created an overly exaggerated, effeminate image of the pimp. And, in turn, many real pimps began to accept and emulate that image of the Hollywood Pimp. Fortunately, today the stereotypical flashy pimp represents a small unit of the pimping world.

Although there are different versions of pimps, and most of them have many different techniques of pimpin', there are some pimpin' rules, laws and standards that are universal. A good pimp will always abide by the basic universal rules of pimpin'. A good pimp is surprisingly sincere. He lives by the adage "be true to the game, and the game will be true to you." A good pimp doesn't have to bullshit his hoes. Once a pimp starts to become dishonest, sneaky and jivey with his girls, he runs the risk of losing them.

If a good pimp has some business or information he wishes not to share with his hoes, instead of him lying to them, he simply tells them to stay out of a pimp's business and everything will be all right. A good pimp never confides in his hoes. That's like parents trying to confide in their children. The pimp has to always remain the authority figure. A good pimp has to always screen for new employees. The old school pimps call this the "cop and blow" method. A pimp has to keep copping new girls for his stable at all times. He never knows when a girl is going to "blow" (leave his stable), so he has to always keep an eye out for new recruits. A good pimp will reject all sexual advances from a ho until she shows him the money. Iceberg Slim called this the "prat out." The prat out is when you display rejection to increase the other person's desire. When a pimp rejects whore, it makes her try that much harder to be accepted. A good pimp will make a ho put down a deposit right away. When people invest in something, they want to be reciprocated.

When the average man takes a woman on a date and spends $20, he expects something in return. When a ho spends $20,000 on a pimp, she *really* wants something in return, and she's not going to want to leave her pimp until she makes good on her investment. All women want a man that they can spoil, treat nice and do things for. The prostitute is not exempt from this, so a pimp is there to satisfy that need.

Pimps and hoes have a very unique relationship. Many prostitutes can pick up a pimp's vibe when she first sees him. This is why many hookers will qualify a potential pimp to see where he is coming from. When a prostitute meets a man in a social setting, she will sometimes act somewhat hostile towards him in order to get a reaction. If she sees any type of fear in his demeanor, she will know that he is a trick or a square. But if the man immediately puts her ass in check, she will know that he may be a bonafide pimp, and she will then try to make him the "chosen one."

Many pimps have ways of spotting true prostitutes in social settings as well. Some prostitutes have little, dysfunctional characteristics that are not easily detected by the untrained eye.

Here is a list of physical characteristics in a woman that suggest she might be a hooker:

*Heavy makeup, especially around the eyes (suggests that she is hiding shame).

*Having a tongue ring, facial piercing or any other forms of self-mutilation (suggests low self-esteem).

*Drug use, especially with the drug ecstasy (sign of co-dependency).

There are other characteristics to look for in a woman's demeanor as well. One characteristic is *overconfidence*. A display of overconfidence suggests that a woman is trying to overcompensate in order to mask some kind of emotional pain. Another common characteristic in a prostitute is **bisexuality.** Women like to have relationships with people who understand them, and who they can be open and honest with. The only person who truly understands the prostitute is a pimp and another hooker. Since there are so few *real* pimps for hoes to choose from, these women have to settle for "relations" with other females like them. This is why the majority of all prostitutes are bisexual or totally lesbian. In perspective, a pimp has to screen, analyze and outthink females at all times.

Here are some basic rules that a good pimp has to remember:

1) A pimp is always right

2) Don't ever let your ho check you.

3) Get your hoes to invest as much as they can as fast as they can. A pimp can't keep a ho forever, and she will "blow" when he least expects it.

4) A good pimp doesn't have to beat on his hoes. If he feels that he needs to get violent with his girls, that means he needs to tighten up his game.

5) Get the money before the "honey." Don't accept sex from your ho until she has reached her quota. Purse first, ass last.

6) Never be at a loss for words.

7) Always keep a cold, serious demeanor with your hoes. Most good pimps rarely smile, because some hoes can take this as a sign of weakness.

8) Your hoes are never equal to you.

9) The more money the ho gives, the longer she stays. So always give yourself a raise.

10) Keep your thoughts a mystery. Never let your hoes know what you are thinking. The more you change your demeanor, the more she will be intrigued with trying to figure you out.

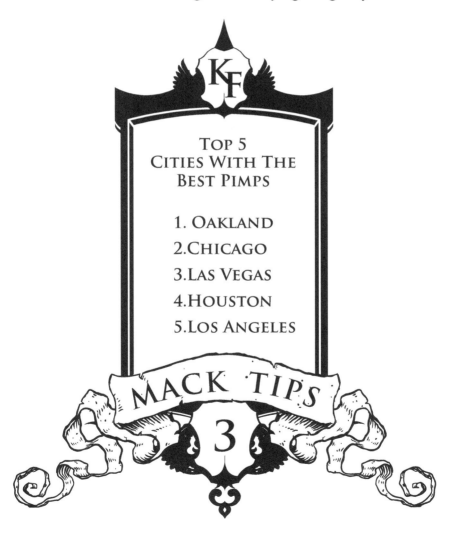

Top 5 Cities With The Best Pimps

1. OAKLAND
2. CHICAGO
3. LAS VEGAS
4. HOUSTON
5. LOS ANGELES

MACK TIPS

3

"A PERSON WHO NEVER MADE A MISTAKE
NEVER TRIED ANYTHING NEW. "

— ALBERT EINSTEIN —

Chapter Four

MACKIN'
DO'S AND DON'TS

By now, you the reader, should have a full understanding of what a true mack is, a general understanding of the type of women out on the dating scene, and an idea of how eextreme Mackin' is put down. Now it's time to learn what makes a true mack tick. There are some general rules that all true macks must abide by.

First and most importantly, one must understand that the essence of a mack is **confidence, confidence,** and **confidence.** Confidence, or a lack thereof, can make or break a mack. Confidence in a person attracts other people to them, and everyone likes to be around a person who seems like a winner. A true mack gives off the impression and demeanor of importance and success, and this is why women are attracted to men like this. When I say giving off the impression of success, that doesn't mean fronting or flossing material items, because doing this shows how much game you don't have.

A man could be the ugliest guy on the block, but if he carries himself like he's "the bomb," essentially people will treat him like he's the bomb. It's hard for many men to find that self-confidence, and this is why many aspiring macks fall by the wayside. There are many factors that contribute to a person having a lack of confidence. The most common reason in men is a fear of rejection. A brother might have had an experience with a woman that he tried to spit game to and she dissed him, so now he has a complex about himself.

Men have to realize that most of the time, when a woman disses you, it's not personal. She may have issues of her own that have nothing to do with you. She may have a boyfriend.She may be living with her baby's daddy.She may be in drug counseling.There could be a number of other reasons that may not permit her to get with any other man at that point in her life.

So, if a woman disses you, instead of second guessing

yourself, look at it as her loss, and move on to the next prospect. A true mack never lets a female knock him off his game. If a professional basketball player has a bad game, he's not going to quit the NBA. He's going to tighten up his skills and play a better game next time.

In order for a brother to become a successful mack, he has to lose the fear of getting dissed. Worrying whether or not you are going to get dissed will stifle your game and cause you to miss out on mackin' opportunities every time. You have to understand that no one is immune to getting dissed. Murphy's Law states that, "If you try to please everybody, somebody won't like it." The simple fact of reality is that some people are going to like you, and some people are not.

Unfortunately, many people tend to focus on the people that don't like them. They often do this because they have an internal need to win approval. What people should realize is that for every two people that don't like you, there are ten people that will jock you. And, in most cases, those two people that don't like you probably don't like anybody. No one is universally loved or hated. It's all about perception. Dr. Martin Luther King, Jr. preached love and equality for all people, and there were individuals who obviously didn't like him or his message of equality, and we've seen the outcome of that. And Pope John Paul, who is considered one of the holiest men in the world and is loved by many, was shot in an assassination attempt during the early 80's. This just goes to show that you could be the nicest, most caring, most saintliest person in the world and there are simply going to be people that just don't feel you.

A mack can have the best looks, the best physique and the best game in the world, but there are going to be some females that are not going to vibe with him. The most important thing is to accept this reality and don't take it personal if you get dissed. Even the finest of women get dissed. Take actress Halle Berry, for example. Halle, who is considered one of the finest sistas in the world, was once on the Oprah show crying about how she almost committed suicide because she got dissed by her ex-husband, baseball player David Justice. Now, jf someone as fine as Halle Berry can get dissed, anyone can. A true mack must have enough confidence and self-esteem to not be thrown off by a dis. There are many ways to build up your confidence and self-esteem. The biggest mistake that people make in general, is when they get into relationships and look to their mate to substantiate their self-worth. People often look for affirmations from others, because they don't find themselves interesting. This is a catch-22, because if you don't find yourself interesting, others won't find you interesting either. Many people have problems with being overly selfcritical. They spend so much time worrying and bellyaching about characteristics that they can't change (for example, "Oh, I have a big forehead"; "My nose is too wide"; or "My penis is too small," etc.). Worrying about things you can't change is a complete waste of time and positive energy. The best thing you can do is concentrate on the things that you can improve, such as getting a new hairstyle; getting better toned at the gym; getting your teeth fixed; improving your wardrobe; going back to school; getting that better job; and other things of that nature. Positive self-improvement is a great selfesteem builder. Sitting around whining and complaining about how people won't accept you because your "ears are too big" is a cop out, and it's used as an excuse to not improve. What if rapper/actor Will Smith sat around worrying if people would accept how big his ears are? Would he be one of the world's biggest box office attractions? Probably not. So, from this point on, stop overemphasizing physical characteristics that you consider "flaws," and start concentrating on your positive traits. There is nothing wrong with giving yourself props.

Start giving positive affirmations to yourself such as, "I have a nice smile. I'm a fun person to be around. I'm smart. My game is tight. I have a nice speaking voice," etc. When you really start to become aware of, and believe in, the positive characteristics that you possess, others will be drawn in by these characteristics as well. When you are giving yourself positive affirmations, avoid using words such as "not" or "I don't," because these are key words that automatically conjure up negative images. So, instead of saying "I'm not ugly" or "I don't act like a buster," say to yourself "I *am* fly" or "My swagger *is* smooth," etc. Those types of affirmations will bring about positive results. Confidence can compensate for unattractiveness. Many women already understand this concept. I was once at a party in Hollywood, and I saw this one young lady who, at first glance, resembled a fruit bat with a weave (and I'm not just making this up). Although this wasn't the most attractive woman in the world, she mingled and walked around that party as if she were Janet Jackson or somebody. And men were stepping to this woman and buying her drinks all night. However way you think of yourself, others will think the same way of you. The great banking tycoon Amshel Rothschild once stated, "If you assume a position of power, people will soon give it to you."

If you carry yourself as if you got it going on, people will treat you like you got it going on. But if you are unsure of yourself, others will be unsure of you as well. Always keep your clothing and grooming habits intact. Our physical appearance has a big influence on the way we carry ourselves. A mack should keep his physical appearance up at all times, and not just on special occasions. Many people who have low self-esteem will fix themselves up maybe once or twice a week to get a confidence boost, and then it's back to the same ol same ol. This is especially particular with women. I often meet women who fix themselves up on the weekend to go out, and they seem almost overconfident. They get their hair and nails done, they have on their best outfits, and they are positive they look the bomb. Some of these women think they are so bomb that they can hardly speak to anybody. These are the women that men claim act snotty or stuck up because of their arrogance and overconfidence. Normally, when you see one of these "overconfident" females during a normal weekday in their personal environment, they are usually back in their slump.

Overconfidence is a sign of insecurity. People who act overconfident feel that they have to over-dramatize a sense of self-esteem in order to make up for their shortcomings. It's good to be confident, because self-assurance *attracts.* However, arrogance and overconfidence *repels.* People who act so into themselves and egotistical turn other people off. All a true mack has to worry about is keeping his body clean, his clothes neat, and his game tight. Another important part about being a mack is having charisma. Having charisma means having an exceptional ability to secure other people's devotion or loyalty. People often think that being a mack means you just spit game at women that you are trying to "screw." But being a charismatic mack means gaining a rapport with all types of women, and forming a genuine friendship with them. This is why it is essential for all macks to have platonic female friends. Many brothers make the mistake of trying to "sex" every woman he knows, but a mack knows that the power of the platonic female friend is underestimated. Platonic female friends are like a "referral service" for macks. If your platonic friend has a homegirl that you want to spit game to, she can give you a rundown on her homegirl's pedigree, and this can save you a lot of mackin' time. Referral hook-ups are considered the most prosperous because people feel more comfortable when they are introduced by a mutual friend.

Another important fact in being a mack is the ability to make women feel comfortable around you. Although you have to be somewhat aggressive in pursuing women, you must also be *smooth* at the same time. Being overly aggressive with women can make them feel pressured, and this will cause them to become defensive and, ultimately, they will be driven away. It is of the uttermost importance that you are smooth, suave and nonthreatening in your demeanor, because this keeps women in a comfort zone.

Women like to hear smooth, and comforting conversation from men, because it gives them a subconscious sense of relaxation. Even if these females realize that a guy is a mack, and that he's kickin' game, they like to hear his conversation anyway because, deep down, it still makes them feel a sense of euphoria.

Many women are attracted to macks because they like the challenge of trying to change him. Whenever a female steps to a guy who is an obvious mack and tries to change him, in the back of her mind she really wants to conquer him. It gives many women a great thrill and a tremendous ego boost to get an untamed player, that other women couldn't train, and turn him into a mild square. But after she conquers this player, the thrill of the chase is now gone, and now she kicks him to the curb. Another rule of mackin' is to settle down on your own recognizance and don't let yourself be trained by female macks. Male macks often attract female macks, and game should always recognize game. Most players do not commit to long-term relationships while they are still in their player stage. As I mentioned earlier, "playin'," for the most part, will only bring you short-term satis- faction, which is not necessarily bad. Some brothers are just not ready for long-term relationships at certain points in their lives. But, even while playing the field, a brother should still possess adequate mackin' skills.

One strategy that a seasoned mack will use on his females (or female), to keep them in check, is to give them the impression that he might commit to one of them, only if she plays her cards right. (The only situation in which I condone this strategy is when a guy is dealing with a female mack or a number of female macks. These types of females want and need to be "played" and "macked.") A good mack never takes a definitive position on an accusation of discrepancy on his part. If a female mack tries to pigeonhole you or push you into a corner for answers or a decision on a particular subject that would jeopardize your mackin' position, you give her an answer that will neither confirm nor deny your true motive or agenda. This helps keep you from *lying* your way out of a situation. Remember, in the mackin' world white lies are fair game, but a seasoned mack doesn't have to lie because he has the ability to *lawyer* his way out of a situation.

Getting Busted

If you are in a relationship with an honest woman, by all means you should be honest and straight up with her as well. But if you are dealing with a female player, you need to stay on top of your game by any means necessary. If you are positive that a female you are dealing with is not stepping to you strictly on an emotional level (and what she really wants is for you to trick off paper or to keep you as her dick on the side), you have every right to play her to the fullest. Let's say one of your female macks has concrete evidence of a discrepancy on your part. (Women like this will always be suspicious of you, because they know that they aren't being straight up.) She may have found a phone number, she may have heard your other woman on the answering machine, or she may have seen you with another woman, etc. The first thing to remember is to *calm down*. Most men have a tendency to put on their "stupid face" whenever they get confronted. This is always a dead giveaway of their guilt. As a mack, you should always turn the tables on *her.*

Let's say your female mack asks you a question like, "Who was that girl I saw you with?" First of all, you have to act like you're offended that she would ever ask you a question like that (all the while not confirming or denying the accusation). Then you totally avoid her question by asking her a series of your own questions (all the while pretending to be more offended) on what exactly is she trying to insinuate. In most cases, when a woman has a feeling that her man is doing something wrong, ninety-five percent (95%) of the time, she's right. But, deep down inside, five percent (5%) of her wants to believe that he's not doing anything wrong. When dealing with a female mack, you should cater to that five percent instinct. Check out the way a square and a true mack would handle the same situation:

Female Mack: "Who was that girl I saw you with?"
Dumb Ass: "What girl?"
Female Mack: "You know what girl I'm talking about, the girl I saw you coming out of the motel with."

Dumb Ass: "Oh, that was just my friend."

Busted! This is how a true mack would handle the same situation:

Female Mack: "Who was that girl I saw you with?"
True Mack: "What do you mean 'Who was that girl you saw me with?' (Acting offended) First of all, why are you coming at me with that accusing tone? (Turning the question on her) Instead of coming to me like an adult (questioning her maturity) and just asking me a question in a respectful way, you're coming at me like I've done something wrong." (Now putting her in the hot seat)
Female Mack: "Well, I'm sorry."
True Mack: "No, what were you trying to insinuate?" (Not letting *her* off the hook)
Female Mack: "Nothing, I just wanted to know who that girl was."
True Mack: "You know what? I'm totally offended, and I don't even want to talk to you about this right now." (Again, totally avoiding the question and mackin' your way out of the situation.)

Notice how the true mack neither confirmed nor denied any wrongdoing. And he did it without telling a lie. Telling lies leads to other lies, plus you have to remember and retrace the lies you have told. This is why it's best to manipulate your words or to be brutally honest with your game, when dealing with a female mack. Notice how the square was actually *answering* the questions. Then he started using the "denial technique." When that didn't work, he simply played dumb, and then straight out lied. Using this type of behavior will get a brother busted by a female mack every time.

To be a mack, you have to shift control of the conversation to yourself. In this way, *you* will be the one asking the questions and demanding answers. Now, I know this may sound somewhat scandalous and deceitfully manipulative, but as I mentioned before, when you are dealing with a female mack you have to play to win. If you don't mack her, she's going to mack you. And I must reiterate that if you are trying to maintain a longlasting and healthy relationship with a female, my advice is to not be dishonest whatsoever. But, even in these types of relationships, there is nothing wrong with using a few mackin' techniques every now and then.

General Mackin' Do's and Don'ts

1).Do have an answer for everything/Don't ever be at a loss for words.

A basic rule of the mackin' game is to never be at a loss for words. To a mack, his verbal skills are his ammunition. When, or if, any situation comes up, you should be able to say the right thing at the right time to rectify the situation. Having a loss of word shows guilt, plus it makes you look stupid to the female. As Rosebudd once said, "If you run out of words, you run out of game."

2).Do have platonic female friends/Don't try to date every woman you know.

As I stated before, you are not going to be compatible with every woman you meet. Some women are going to have a different agenda than yours. If a female is looking for a brother to help pay some of her bills, no matter how good you look, or how tight your game is, if you're not tricking off any money, she's not interested in a relationship with you. In cases like this, don't blow her off completely. Just put her in the platonic zone. As a platonic friend, she can hook you up with her other friends, all the while giving you the 411 on them.

3).Do carry yourself like a real man at all times/Don't act overly emotional or overly sensitive.

One of the biggest complaints women have about men is that many of them don't have any backbone. Too many men are acting emotional and overly sensitive with women. And when they do, women often accuse these men of "acting like bitches." As a mack, you let your emotions remain a mystery, and always keep your composure. As a mack, you should generally have a nonchalant attitude. Your demeanor should basically be casual and unconcerned. This will keep women intrigued and trying to figure out what your feelings are and what you are thinking. However, women will lose that intrigue if you reveal your feelings by acting overly emotional or jealous. Jealousy is a sign of insecurity. Many times, women will test your "jealousy meter" to see how you will react. If a woman says something like "There's this guy at work that likes me," or "My ex' called, and he wants me to meet him for a drink. What should I do?" or something of that nature, it's a test. You have to let her know that you are so confident with yourself, and your game is so tight, it would be ridiculous for her to even think of stepping to the next man. Your demeanor is that you really don't care what she does, and at this point she will put herself in check. But you should never rant, rage and act jealous, because a female will then consider you a buster.

4).Do learn how to read women/Don't assume you know everything about women.

The only people that come close to knowing almost everything about women are seasoned macks and seasoned pimps. (Many women don't know everything about themselves.) A lot of untrained, aspiring macks step to women thinking they know everything, and then end up getting played. A lot of brothers think that mackin' is just stepping to women and spitting out a bunch of cliche pickup lines. This is how you get dissed. The key to having good game is to **mack, then react**.

A lot of men will start kicking game to a female, and continue to kick game, even if she's not showing any interest whatsoever. This is a waste of valuable mackin' time. A mack will step to a female and kick some opening game to break the ice. Then he will kick back for a second to watch her reaction. And most of the time, he is not only listening to what she is saying, he is also looking at and reading her body language. From her reaction to his opening game, the mack will then counter-react, so on and so forth. (More on the mack and react techniques in the next chapter.)

To be a good mack, you have to learn how women think. Many women seem to suppress their true motives and agendas when communicating with men, but they tend to be very open and honest with each other. So not only should you listen to what women say to you, listen and pay attention to what women say to each other. Read an issue of Essence magazine, watch the Oprah Show, or check out the Lifetime channel every now and then to give yourself an idea of how women think and react. This, in turn, will help you understand and deal with women more knowledgeably.

Another way of getting an angle on a female is to learn information about her ex. When you first meet females, they try to portray themselves in the most attractive way possible, so they are less likely to reveal any faults or misgivings. But once you get into a comfort zone with them, and ask them questions about their ex, they are more than willing to dish out all of the dirt on his negative qualities. In many cases, all the negative qualities applied to the ex man can be applied to the female as well, because people tend to date those who are reflections of themselves. So if a woman says that her ex-boyfriend was a "lowbudget, crackhead that sat around and didn't want to work," what does that say about her since she chose to date him? In most cases, only a lowbudget woman will date a low-budget man.

5).Do keep up your appearance/Don't floss and front.

As I mentioned earlier, you don't have to be a baller to look like one. For a true mack, proper hygiene is not an option; it's a necessity. And you don't have to have on the most expensive clothes to look *neat.* (Don't run out and buy a $200 Versace shirt, and then wear it every other day.) The first thing a woman looks at, appearancewise, is a man's shoes, so make sure your footwear is up to par. Confidence in your appearance will make you more confident in your attitude. It's hard to have confidence in yourself when you are worrying if your green cowboy boots look right with your red jumpsuit. When your clothes are screaming for attention, it's a sign of you having no game. Wearing a bunch of gaudy jewelry is played, and bragging about material items (especially if you don't have any) makes you look like a buster. Women like men whose game can speak for itself.

6).Do realize that as a mack, you deserve the best/ Don't ever "trick off your money.

Don't be afraid to mack up on the best women on the market. A lot of times when a square brother does luck up on an overly fine or top-notch sista, he starts to second-guess himself. He starts to think to himself, "If a girl this fine is with me, then something must be wrong with her." Or he will begin to feel insecure, and will assume that if she finds out his true persona, she is going to dump him for someone better. This causes him to subconsciously sabotage the relationship and, eventually, the relationship will sever. Also, in cases such as this, the square will feel like he has to trick off his money just to keep the female, and this causes her to lose respect for him.

Here's another important rule of the mackin' game. No matter how fine a woman is, do not make it seem as if she's doing you a favor by being with you. Make it seem like she should be privileged to be in the presence of a mack such as yourself. Don't ever jock a female. This shows signs of desperation, which in turn, shows signs of insecurity and a need for attachment. Don't be a bug-a-boo, calling a woman on the phone three and four times a day, unless it's mutual. If you call a woman more than three times on three separate occasions, and she rushes off the phone and never calls you back, toss her number to the curb, because more than likely she considers you to be a bug-a-boo. Continuing to call her is only making it worse. Instead of wasting valuable phone and mackin' time on someone who isn't reciprocating, you could be stepping to other females who are more compatible and receptive to your game.

One of the most important things for an aspiring mack to remember is that a true mack never tricks off his paper. Doing this on a regular basis will cause your T.M.A. membership to be revoked. The only time a mack spends his money on a female is when he is on a date or if the female is his significant other. But spending money on a female (like paying her rent, paying for salon trips, paying her bills, etc.) when the female is **not** your lady, automatically takes you out of the mackin' category and sends you straight to trick status.

There are many titles for guys that spend money on females in order to compensate for a lack of game. Some of the most common titles are "simp," "sugar daddy," "captain save-a-ho," etc. But all of these names lead to one title: *trick.* And the trick is the antithesis to the mack.

7).Do use tact/Don't be argumentative.

A good mack always has to use tact when kicking game. Remember, you must have the ability to do and say the right thing at the right time. Some guys step to all females the same way, and this is why they end up getting dissed most of the time. Your game has to be flexible. You have to tailor your game to the type of female you're mackin' to.

For example, if you were to step to the average top-notch female, your demeanor should be more on the straightforward and aggressive side. This is because most topnotch females are used to having an intimidating affect on men, so they need a man who isn't afraid to stand up to them.

Now, the middle-class girl (the homegirl) has more of a laid back, family-oriented, nurturing disposition. So she would be more receptive to the warmer, "sweet mackin'" approach. Coming at her with the straightforward, aggressive approach would more than likely drive her away. This is why you must have the ability to change up your game when it's appropriate. A lot of men step to females by saying anything that comes to mind, no matter how insulting it is. These guys justify it by claiming they are "keeping it real." Being real doesn't mean that you have to be **rude.** Always have discretion and diplomacy in your game, because rudeness and belligerence show that you may be trying to cover up your own insecurities, and you feel the need to tear down others to build yourself up. Granted, there are some females that won't give you the time of day unless you are cursing them out or stepping to them in hardcore pimp mode. But you can't step to every female like this.

Another thing that a true mack doesn't do is argue with women. Arguing is oftentimes a result of losing your composure and emotions, and a true mack should be calm, cool and composed at all times. Theoretically, arguing is usually a healthy part of normal relationships, because it helps couples determine what buttons to push and which ones not to push. It shows couples what could trigger each other's anger, and it helps give options to settle differences. But, as a mack, you have to let it be known that a female shouldn't even **think** about trying to push any of your buttons. Squares **argue,** but macks put women in *check.* A mack says what he wants to say, and he leaves it at that. If a female tries to lure a mack into an argument, he doesn't take the bait. He lets her know that if she can't discuss the issues in a calm manner, like an adult, then there is nothing to discuss. Case closed.

It's also important to note that a true mack never "lies on his dick." Going around bragging about how many females you've slept with, when you really haven't, makes you look like a buster. This causes you to lose T.M.A. points as well. A true mack is secure enough in his game to admit that he may be having difficulties with getting the draws from a particular female. Everyone is subject to human error, and a brother who "fronts" like every female is on his jock is not being true to the game.

Now that you have a basic understanding of the mackin' do's and don'ts, you are ready to test your mackin' skills. But, first, let's review *the 20 general rules of mackin'*:

1). Always have confidence.

2). Always keep up your appearance.

3). Never "lie on your dick."

4). Don't talk too much.

5). Always appear to be calm and relaxed.

6). Don't ever dwell on getting "dissed," it happens to the best of us.

7). Never be at a loss for words.

8). Always have platonic female friends.

9). Never pay for sex.

10). Keep your demeanor as emotionless as possible.

11). Listen more to a woman's nonverbal language.

12).Never fight with another man if your lady chooses him.

13). Always keep new females coming into your fold.

14). Don't front or act overly flossy.

15). Don't be a bug-a-boo.

16). Don't argue with women.

17). Never let women figure you out.

18). Never seem overly anxious when you're hooking up with a female.

19). Never hit women.

20). Never, ever, ever trick off your money.

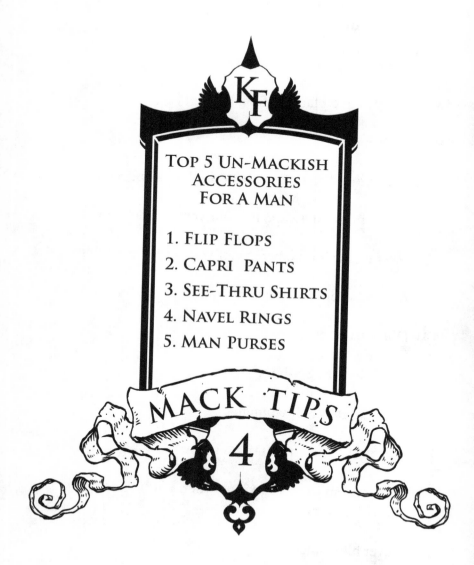

Top 5 Un-Mackish
Accessories
For A Man

1. Flip Flops
2. Capri Pants
3. See-Thru Shirts
4. Navel Rings
5. Man Purses

MACK TIPS

4

"BECOMING A MAN DOESN'T MEAN
REACHING A CERTAIN AGE, IT
MEANS REACHING A CERTAIN
STATE OF MIND."

— ASHLEY BERG —

Chapter Five

HOW TO WORK THE CLUB

Now that you have an understanding of all the mackin' do's and don'ts, it is time for you to step into the mackin' arena. The nightclub, to a mack, is what a NBA player is to a basketball court, what a lion is to a jungle, and what a NFL player is to a football field. In the square world, the nightclub is considered the least desirable place to seek out a long-term and healthy relationship. But in the mackin' community, the club is a mack's natural habitat. As I mentioned previously, playing the field generally produces short-term fulfillment, and what better place to satisfy those short-term needs than a nightclub?

One of the reasons it is considered so hard (but not impossible) to get into a lasting relationship with someone you meet at a club is because people tend to get into a "club mode" when they go out on the weekends. When people get into club mode, they do things they normally wouldn't do on a regular, daily basis or "natural mode." When people go to clubs, they wear things they wouldn't normally wear on a regular weekday. They wear their hair in a style that they normally don't wear on a daily basis. They wear certain makeup that they normally wouldn't wear on a daily basis. They sometimes drive cars (rented Bentleys and Lexuses) that they normally don't drive on a daily basis.

So, in most cases, when you meet a person at a club, you become interested in their club persona. But when you get to see them outside of a club setting and in their natural setting, you might see that she doesn't look good without makeup; her weave is looking raggedy; her home is torn up; she drives a bucket; or any one of a dozen things that make you lose interest. In order to find a relationship with any real significance, it's best to meet people in their normal everyday surroundings. Places like the supermarket, the laundromat, the post office, the gym or any other public place where people generally feel like they don't have to put on any fronts are the best places for a possible long-term hook-up. But when you're going through a player stage in your life, the club is the premiere place to satisfy your needs.

In this chapter, I will show some tried and proven ways to

pick up women in clubs. I will show you how to screen for women who may become your next potential prey. I will also tell you what to do and say to get women to leave the club with you. Most men have one ultimate goal in mind when they go out to clubs.

That goal is to meet a female, take her home, and hit that ass. Some men will *settle* for just a phone number or just having a dance, a drink or some social conversation with a woman, but what he really wants to do is to mack up on some ass for the night. So, for the sake of this chapter, we will assume that your goal is to mack a woman up out of the club. This is how a mack would go about it, and this is what you should do.

Prepare Your Allies

When you go out to the club, you should have at least one to two other homies with you. For one, you feel more comfortable and confident when you go out with other people. Going out by yourself can put on added pressure if you're not a seasoned mack. Plus, when you go out with at least two other homies, you can have one act as a checkmate and the other as a scavenger.

Oftentimes, when you step to a female (the prey) in a club,

and she is with a friend that is as equally fine as her (the salt shaker), the friend will often try to throw salt in your game. The main reason she does this is that you didn't step to her instead. This is why you have to hook the salt shaker up with your checkmate homey.

In the game of chess, when you checkmate an opponent, you make it so that no defense is possible. So, when you hook the checkmate homey up with the salt shaking female, you do this to keep her preoccupied from throwing salt in your game. This is important, because if you are trying to mack to your potential prey, and she has a salt shaker with her (and you don't have a checkmate with you), the salt shaker is going to start cockblocking your game. The salt shaker will do things such as grabbing her friend's hand and saying, "C'mon, girl, let's go to the ladies room" or "Let's go over to the bar," all the while throwing a wrench in your game.

Now, if you step to a female who has a not-so- desirable friend with her (the buzzard), this is where your scavenger homey comes into play. All men have at least one homey that will bone *anything.* The definition of a scavenger is "one who searches for something useful in discarded material," and that is what the "scavenger" homey does. He will take the female that nobody else wants. This is why it is helpful to take the checkmate and the scavenger homey out with you to the clubs.

Scout Your Territory

When you walk into a club, you have to think of yourself as a lion out on the plains of Africa. Before you attack your prey, you have to become familiar with the terrain. When you arrive at a club, you have to sit back in the "cut" and observe the women around you. You must get a feel of the *vibe* in the club. You must also get an idea of the types of women that are in the club.

From my observations over the years, I've noticed that women usually go out in cliques of two's and four's. Many women do go out by themselves, but it is more common for them to go out in groups because they feel more comfortable in the presence of friends. Since your goal is to mack a female up out of the club, it's best to spit at a female who is rollin' solo or a female who has only one other female friend with her.

Although it is highly possible to pull a female who is in a group of four, you want to go for the best odds possible, and reduce the amount of salt shakers that might cockblock your game. (In reference to this chapter, the term "pull" means to get a female to leave the club with you.)

Don't waste your time trying to pull a female who is in a group of five or more, because when there are that many females in a group, they are usually visiting from out of town or something of that nature, and these females feel that they have to stick together at all times. Plus, when it's a group that large, they probably drove to the club in two or more separate vehicles, and that's a complex situation within itself. So it's best to try to pull females who are in groups of four or less. Women that go out in groups of four generally get along with each other because they have four different personalities. It's often hard for women to get along with one another when they are equal in beauty and personality, because this often creates jealousy, competitiveness and combativeness. So, in order for a group of females to click with one another, they all have to vary in their demeanor.

Normally, when females go out to clubs in groups of four, you have:

1).The Smart One
2).The Ho'ish One
3).The Ding'y One
4).The Buzzard

These women can be any one of the "4 H's," but some of them can lean more towards a specific "H" than others. Here is a rundown of all four girls and which ones to talk to:

The Smart One

The smart one is usually the ringleader of the group. She is usually the most intelligent one in the group, and the rest of the girls pretty much do whatever she says. In many cases, this female would also fall into the top-notch or middle- class girl category. The smart one is usually the best one to try to pull out of a group of four. This is because she is the type of female that is used to making her own decisions and she doesn't buckle under to peer pressure from her friends.

The Ho'ish One

Since this type of female comes to the club dressed all hoochie (with her cleavage showing and her ass hanging out) and acting stank (by dancing real freaky, rubbing up on guys, and shaking her ass wildly), a lot of men think that she is easy prey. Nothing can be further from the truth. Notice when describing this female, I used the term "ho'ish" not "ho." In many cases, this female is not technically a ho, but she acts like one in order to get attention. Oftentimes, this female falls into the ghetto queen (hoodrat) or the rebound chick category.

She may be in a vicinity relationship or she may be feeling insecure because she is on bad terms with her man. So she dresses up as hoochie as possible, goes to the club with her friends, and carries on like a stank ho. These females hardly ever give up the ass.

They figure that, since they aren't having sex with guys besides their boyfriends (or husbands), they can go out and act as ho'ish as possible. They justify their overly stank disposition by reasoning that they are "just having fun" and "it's not like I'm fucking these guys," etc.

The only intention of the ho'ish female is to have guys ogle over her in efforts to boost her sabotaged ego. When that is accomplished, she's going straight home to her man. So trying to pull the ho'ish one out of a group of girls in a club is, in most cases, a huge waste of time (though it is not impossible). And since every other guy in the club thinks she is easy prey, they have all put their bids in, and now her superficial ego is erroneously blown way out of proportion. Now she thinks she is all that, and as I mentioned earlier, some women forge this type of overconfidence in order to mask their insecurities.

The Ding'y One

The ding'y one is almost child-like in her demeanor. She just likes to tag along with her friends and do whatever they tell her to do. In many cases, the ding'y one is the non-Black female out of the group. The ding'y one acts like she can't do anything without the intervention of her friends. If you ask her to dance, or to come over to the VIP room, she'll say something like, "My friends don't have nobody to dance with" or "I don't want to leave my friends."

In many instances, you'll see the ding'y girl's friends literally holding her hand and leading her around the club like she's a kid. Although it is somewhat difficult to pull a **ding'y** girl out of the club, it is not impossible. The key thing is, you have to separate her from the group.

On the plains of Africa, the stronger antelope will often herd around and shield the weaker antelope in order to protect it from the lions. You have to get the ding'y girl alone and away from the "herd," so you can then launch your mack attack. Once you've gotten the ding'y one in your zone, you need to put a checkmate homey on the smart one so she won't try to throw salt in your game.

The Buzzard

The buzzard female may not be necessarily ugly, but she is considered the least desirable one out of the group. She might be a little less attractive or a little more overweight than the other girls, and they bring her along to balance out the clique. (In many cases the buzzard is the one driving.) The buzzard usually has a major attitude because the guys in the club are talking to her friends and not her. She's also the one complaining all night about how she's not having a good time, and how much she's "ready to go." All these factors cause her to be an avid salt shaker.

If you try to talk to one of her friends, you have to immediately hook her up with your scavenger homey, so she won't get a chance to cockblock your game. The buzzard, by definition, is a scavenger as well, so this female is a perfect match for your scavenger homey.

When you walk into a club, you have to mingle before you mack. When you are screening for females to pull out of the club, you have to be very observant. There are some chickenheads who disguise themselves as middle-class girls and there are some hoodrats who disguise themselves as topnotch. You should be wary of the ghetto queens and chickenheads because they usually have a bunch of kids that need to be picked up from the baby-sitter, or they have a man that they have to go home to. So you are less likely to pull one of them out of the club.

Also, stay away from the liquor hustlers. Liquor hustlers are females who hang out by the bar and flirt with men in order to get free drinks. Although it is acceptable to purchase drinks for women in clubs, a truly seasoned mack never buys women drinks. If he has to buy a woman a drink just to break the ice, that means his game isn't tight enough.

Buying females drinks in clubs often has trick overtones, and a mack doesn't come off like a trick whatsoever. Also, watch out for underage girls who use fake IDs to get into clubs. You can often tell if a female is underage by the way she walks. In many cases, these women are not used to high-heeled shoes, and when they wear them, they tend to stomp down hard and awkwardly when walking. Also, if you start a conversation with these females, and they sound ghetto and immature, that's usually a dead giveaway.

Also, watch out for flamboyant Asian, White and Hispanic girls who hang out in predominantly Black clubs, because more than likely, these girls are groupies. These girls figure that, if they are going home with a Black guy, he is going to be a sports, television, recording or movie star. You can step to these women with the best game in the world, but if you're not a celebrity, they're not feeling you. So don't trip on them.

Surprisingly, the easiest females to pull out of the club are the top-notch females (especially if she's rollin' solo). Also, it's easy to pull two of the five dysfunctional types of females (the rebound chick and the sanctified, shy girl) as well.

As I mentioned before, guys often try to pull loose and flashy women that are running around the club acting stank. But it's the quiet, conservative female sitting off in the corner that will more than likely leave the club with you. For one, she is more receptive to companionship because she is in a public place by herself, and her defenses are not as high as the other females in the club. If she's an overly fine, top-notch female, she's open to be macked because most guys are intimidated by her and they figure that she won't give them the time of day. If she's a rebound chick or an overly shy girl, most likely she's emotionally vulnerable, and this makes her easy prey.

Mastering Your Approach

As I stated earlier, the essence of a mack is confidence. One way to maintain your confidence when you go to a club is to carry yourself as if you are an important person (this doesn't mean frontin' and flossin'). If you act as if you are an important person, people will treat you as if you are important. One way to do this is by using visualization. Imagine yourself as being the owner of the club. Think about how the owner of the club would carry himself and how he would mingle with the patrons. Would the owner of the club walk around flossin' and frontin'? Probably not, because he's runnin' things and he has no need to front. Would he be confident and charismatic with the clubgoers? Yes, he would, because he wants his patrons to be comfortable and to have a good time. So, if you *carry* yourself as if you were runnin' things (without *fronting* like you are runnin' things), people will treat you as such.

It's also important that you don't rely solely on alcohol for the confidence you need. Alcohol is cool if you just want to loosen up, but you shouldn't go overboard. Alcoholic beverages seem to give you courage because it removes inhibitions. But, in most cases, it also removes tactfulness, and this can cause some brothers to come off like assholes once they've had one too many drinks.

Now, when you step to a female, your tone and demeanor have to be correct. This is called getting into mack mode. When you're mackin' to a female, don't talk too loud or too fast. Oftentimes, in a club you have to talk loud because of the music volume, but you should still try to control your voice volume as much as possible. Fast talking is a sign of nervousness, and women can sense this. You have to talk to a woman very *slowly* while making direct eye contact with her. This puts you in an authoritative position over the female, and it shows that you are confident in what you are saying. Also, when you talk slow, your voice automatically gets deeper, thus adding more authority to your tone. When you are mackin', your voice has to sound soothing and melodic, almost putting the female in a hypnotic state. When a female is in this "semi-altered, almost hypnotic state," her mind is more receptive to your commands.

Another key thing to remember when you're in mack mode is, never *ask* a woman to do something. You should always *instruct* her to do it. When you ask a female to do something, this puts her in a position over you, and you give her the option to say no. So, instead of *asking* a female at a club, "Would you like to dance?"; "Can I have your phone number?"; or "Do you want to sit down and talk?" you *tell* her to "Come dance with me"; "Write your number down"; or "Come sit down and talk with me." This shows women that you are confident enough to be direct, and man enough to take the initiative in a situation.

Breaking the Ice

Now, a lot of guys have trouble approaching females with an opening line. Your opening line should never sound contrived or cliche, because most females can tell when a brother is using a concocted pickup line. When you step to females, your game has to make them feel comfortable. A lot of women walk around the club with their defenses up because so many lame brothers have been trying to kick weak game to them. Your approach has to be interesting to the point where she would want to let her guards down, so your opening line has to sound natural and appropriate for the situation.

There are **four basic ways for a mack to approach a female**. He can use:

1). The humorous approach
2). The innocent approach
3). The direct mack approach; or
4). The go-for-broke approach.

When using the *humorous approach,* it's best to be clever and witty, but not too silly. Most women like men with a sense of humor, so if you can put a smile on a woman's face by stepping to her with something innovative and different, you will at least get your foot in the door. There is no *one* line that will work on all females, because every woman is different in her own way.

This is why a mack has to be spontaneous. Over the years, I've used thousands of opening lines on various women. Usually, these are lines that I just make up on the spot. The females were receptive to my opening lines because they were sincere and not contrived.

Here is an example of how you can step to a female by using the humorous approach:

Mack: "Y'know, I have a dozen pickup lines that I wanna use on you. Which ones do you wanna hear first?" (You have to say this in a tongue-in-cheek sort of way.)

Female: "Let me hear what you got."

Mack: "Okay, here we go ... 'What's a nice girl like you doing in a place like this?'; 'What's your sign?'; 'Do you come here often?'; 'I drive a Benz.'; 'I play for the Clippers.'; i 'm a bodyguard for Gary Coleman.' So, are you impressed with any of these lines yet?"

If the female is somewhat intelligent, she will understand that the "mack" is being delightfully sarcastic, and that his opening line is basically a goof on guys who actually use those lines seriously.

By using the humorous approach, you can say anything that comes to mind, as long as it is tactful.

And remember to not worry about getting dissed. This is where the slot machine mentality comes into play. If you get dissed, you have to keep on playing until you hit the jackpot.

The humorous approach is more effective when used on top-notch and some middleclass females. These types of females are also more receptive to the innocent approach than other females. By using this approach, you don't step to the female in an overly direct manner, but more in an innocently casual sort of way. You would say something to the effect of, "Have you been to this club before? (She gives her response and you continue) Well, this is my first time here, and I feel kind of strange because I'm unfamiliar with the crowd and the atmosphere." (This shows her that you are confident enough within yourself that you can admit your discomfort. This also makes her lower her defenses.) Then you would proceed to say, "So, what do you know about this club?" (This causes her to reply, plus it makes you appear to be nonthreatening, so she lowers her defenses even more.) The female may reply with something like, "I've only been here a few times myself, and I don't know too much about the crowd here either."

Then you would switch back into mack mode and spit game at her like, "Well, the reason I came up to ask you is that you're one of the few decent-looking females in here." Now, this line is very effective, because the average fine sista in a club thinks that she looks better than the next chick. So, even if she realizes that you are kickin' game" to her, her natural competitiveness causes her to believe that she is one of the most (if not the most) decent-looking females in the club.

The reason that the humorous and innocent approaches work best on high-class sistas and homegirls is because these women are generally confident with themselves. They don't need a guy to floss and trick off drinks for them, because they can buy their own drinks. All they want is a man who can step to them with some decent conversation.

On the other hand, when mackin' to a hoodrat or a chickenhead, you have to use the direct mackin' approach. A lot of these socalled ghetto girls won't even respect a man unless he's coming at them hard-core. A lot of these types of females will take politeness for weakness, and they tend to go around the club screening for tricks. The only man that a ghetto girl will deal with in a club is a pushover who is tricking off drinks and dollars, or a direct mack that is not intimidated by the rigid persona these females project. With the direct mackin' approach, you have to almost get into pimp mode. You must keep an emotionless expression on your face, and only speak when you are giving her a command, or asking her a specific question. Don't engage in any small talk with her. You have to let your persona remain a mystery to her. You must also use a lot of nonverbal communication with her, like giving her the "sexy player eyes," and the enticing licking of the lips. (In a masculine way) your facial expression should say, "You know you wanna 'get boned' tonight."

You must also stay in control of the conversation with these types of females. Since many of these hoodrats and chickenheads (ghetto girls) usually come from single-parent homes where they were primarily raised by their mothers, they are subconsciously looking for that father figure in a man. This is why you have to be direct with them to the point where you are almost talking to them as if they were children. These women are looking for "male direction" and you, as a mack, should provide that direction.

Although pulling a female that is visiting from out of town out of a club is a long shot, like I mentioned earlier, it is not impossible. When spitting game to a female out-of-towner, you have to use the go-for-broke approach. Since she is only going to be in town temporarily, and more than likely you will never see her again, you can immediately cut to the chase and go in for the kill. This is how you work it. (Trust me; this has worked many times before.) You step to her and say, "Look, you're leaving back out of town tomorrow, right?" (In most cases, if it's a female's last night in a city, she probably wants to go out and get buck wild before she leaves anyway.) She may reply, "Yes, this is my last night here. Why?" Then you come at her like this: "Since this is your last night in town, you and I need to get out of here and kick it at my place tonight." I know that may sound a little over-the-top, but I have actually said this to females, and it has worked. You would be surprised at how many females would go along with you, just on the fact that you had the balls (and the confidence) to come at them like that.

If, by chance, she does get offended by this approach, so what? You two will never see each other again anyway, so you have nothing to lose and ass to gain. (By the way, this strategy works particularly well on hoodrats.) You'll also be surprised at how many females have a secret desire to go out of town, meet a stranger, get freaky with him, and go back home to their normal lives. This is one reason why spring break events (such as Freaknik, Mardi Gras, etc.) are so popular. Every year, thousands of females flock to certain cities for spring break, and do all types of outrageous things that they wouldn't normally do in their hometowns. And when spring break is over, these females go back home as if nothing ever happened.

Since I have shown you some of the most common mackin' approaches you should use, here are the **top six opening lines that you should *never* use:**

1)."You got a man?"
2)."Can I get to know you?"
3)."You so fine, I had to come over and say something to you."
4)."Can I get you a drink?"
5)."What yo name is?"
6)."Don't I know you?"

These lame pickup lines generally don't work because females know that they are not *personal*. Most females know that these lines are preconceived, and that they were probably used on every other female in the club. This is why your opening line has to fit that particular female's persona, because women hate to be lumped into a category with every other woman.

Another thing to remember is that your conversation with a female has to last at least three minutes if you're trying to pull, or even to get a phone number. You can't just step to a female and say, "What's your name?" or "Let me get your number." This shows that you have been stepping to females like this all night, and you really don't want to get to know *her*. Basically, you haven't given her a reason to give you her number. Always use the three-minute mackin' technique, because this helps you gain a rapport with the female, and it lowers her defenses.

As I mentioned earlier, it is very important for you to know how to read body language, because some brothers that are unable to read nonverbal signals end up hanging around females so long that they become pests. If a female gives you brief or one-word answers to your questions, this is a sign of her being disinterested. When a female *leans in* to ask or answer a question, this is a sign of interest. But if you find yourself leaning in towards her to ask questions, this is a sign of her being disinterested.

Females crossing their arms or their legs while standing is a sign of insecurity. Many females that have complexes about their stomachs being too big or flabby often cross their arms *low* in order to hide their bellies. And women who are insecure about their breasts often cross their arms higher in order to cover their chest. Women who have a complex about their toes will cross their legs or fold their feet over each other if they feel that someone is watching their shoes. Looking for weaknesses and insecurities such as these will help you determine which females are vulnerable enough for the pull. You should also be watchful of females who talk to you in a high-pitched, childlike voice, while batting their eyes, because this is a sign of deceit. These women may be liquor hustlers that are just trying to sweet-talk you into buying them drinks, so peep game.

Here is an example of one of the most common techniques I've used to pull women out of clubs. First, I would scope the club for prospects and give them a visual evaluation. If I saw a female that I liked, I would scope her out to see if she was with a crowd of five or more; if she were, she'd be scratched. I would also screen females to see if they were ghetto or not. Girls who walk around the club with dollar bills taped to their chests, claiming "It's my birthday," are ghetto. Girls who walk around the club with no shoes on are ghetto. (This implies that she is used to wearing high-heeled shoes only one day a week, and she can barely do that.) Once I see that a female is ghetto, she gets scratched as well because, as I mentioned earlier, these females have other issues to deal with.

My main goal would be to get a middleclass girl, or a top-notch girl who is riding solo. Let's say I was to spot two potential prospects. Before I would go into full-fledged mack mode, I would just sprinkle a little game on them to plant the seed of the actual pull. I would walk up to the first girl and ask, "What's your name?" Hypothetically, she may reply, "Kim. What's your name?" Then I might say, "My name is Tariq. Look, Kim, when they play a song that I like, I want you to dance with me." Her reply would be, "Okay, that'll work," or something to that extent. Then, I'll just walk away. (Notice how I made it seem that if we dance, it can only be on my terms. This puts me in an authoritative position over her.) By doing this, I plant the seed for intrigue to build up.

When the average guy steps to a female and just starts mackin' right away, the female knows that either he wants a phone number or he wants sex (or her phone number *and* sex). This approach turns females off, because there was no smoothness to it. But by using the "seed planting" approach, you keep your true agenda a mystery, and this sparks interest in the female's mind. Since she doesn't have an *angle* on you, a lot of thoughts go on in the back of her mind ("Is he really interested? Is he really waiting for his song to come on? Does he have someone better to talk to?" etc.). This, in turn, causes her to be more interested in you. At this point, I would then proceed to prospect number two.

A quick note to remember here is to work opposite sides of the room one at a time. That means if you mack to one female, don't mack to the one that's two feet away from her. Always go to the other side of the room and "work" the prospects there. Once a female is interested in you, she is going to be keeping an eye on you and peeping your game. So the last thing you want to do is salt yourself. Now, when I step to prospect number two, on the opposite side of the room, I plant the same seed with her, just like I did with girl number one. When I decide to step to these females a second time, it seems that I have somewhat of a rapport with them, because now I know them on a first-name basis. This makes women feel more comfortable.

When I step to girl number one (Kim) again, I purposely use her name a lot during conversation. By using a person's name frequently during conversation, this makes them feel more special and appreciated, and it also makes them more receptive to your game. I would step to girl "number one" and say something like, "Whassup, Kim, you having a good time so far?" etc. After her response, I would take control of the situation by saying, "C'mon, Kim, we're going to go over here and sit down so we can talk." (Notice I didn't ask, I *instructed*.) This is also a good screening process. For example, f she says something like, "My friends are standing here and I don't want to leave them," this probably means that she is one of the ding'y girls I mentioned earlier, and you don't want to mack to her anyway. And if she says something like "Well, I was on my way to the bar," that would suggest that she is a chickenhead liquor hustler, and you don't want to mack to her either. In most cases, a female who is down with your game will follow your lead. And when she does, that means you have your foot in the door.

At this point a lot of men salt themselves, because after they've gotten their foot in the door with a successful approach, they don't know how to keep their game going. The key to keeping a decent conversation going with a female is to get her to talk about herself. The way I do this depends on her physical characteristics. If her attire is somewhat conservative, I'll say something like, "You look like you could be a school teacher or a nurse, or maybe an administrative worker, or something like that. What do you do for a living?" Or if she looks physically fit, I would say, "You look like you could be a personal trainer or a Tae-Bo instructor. What do you do?" (This is also a subtle way of giving her a compliment without sounding like you're brown-nosing her.) Ass-kissing compliments such as "Girl, you so fine" and "You are so sexy" make you come off like a buster. Now, if she says, "Yes, I'm a school teacher. How did you guess?" I would get her to elaborate more by replying to her, "Well, you look very educated. So, where do you teach?" etc. Even if she's not a teacher or a nurse, she will most likely correct you on what her real occupation is. (She may say something like, "I'm not a teacher, but I do work with children, because I'm a counselor," etc.) Then you get her to elaborate on that. When a woman is comfortable enough to talk to you about her personal life, this is a good indication that your game is working. If the conversation goes past the three-minute mackin' time frame, this means your game is working well. Females know within the first few minutes of meeting a man whether she wants to have sex with him or not. All you have to do is not mess it up.

Once you get your foot in the door with a female, it's important that you use seductive and suggestive body language with her ("player eyes," deep, slow voice, etc.) and not talk too much. Now, it's time to go in for the kill. At this point, I would say to the female, "Look, Kim, who did you come here with?" She may reply, "By myself or "With my friend." Then I would continue to screen her by asking, "So, what are you doing when you leave here tonight?" Most likely she will respond, "I was planning on going home and going to bed." (Now, don't be thrown by this answer. This is her way of giving *you* the opportunity to "mack her out of the club." You're still on the right track.) If she replies, "I don't know. Why?" you're *definitely* on the right track. Then, I would proceed with "Look, check this out, Kim. You're gonna go to breakfast with me tonight. What time do you have right now?" Notice how, after the first suggestion, I don't even give her the option to say yes or no. And by asking the follow-up question, "What time do you have now?" I've already made the assumption that we are leaving together, and now all we have to do is establish a time frame. Let's say she tells me, "It's 1:30 right now." Then I would say, "I want you to meet me by the front door in 15 minutes, then we are gonna roll out, okay?" Now, if your game has been tight throughout the evening, then she's gonna be like, "Okay, cool." It's also important to note that the term "Let's go to breakfast" is a euphemism for "Let's go have sex." I've been using the "Let's go to breakfast" line on females in clubs for years, and when I've left the club with them, I have yet to have an actual meal. Also, just as a precaution, you should step to any other prospective females in the club and use the same pulling technique on them as well. A good mack always has a backup plan, just in case the first prospect falls through. The pull is not a done deal until the female walks out of that door with you. If the female is rolling solo, then you're pretty much home free. But if she has a friend (or friends) with her, you need to pull her out of the club as soon as possible.

Eighty percent (80%) of all pulls are foiled because of a salt-shaking-ass friend, who is trying to cockblock your game. But if you use the techniques that I have shown you in this chapter, you should have no problems with pulling a female out of a club. Now all you have to worry about is handling your business like a real mack should.

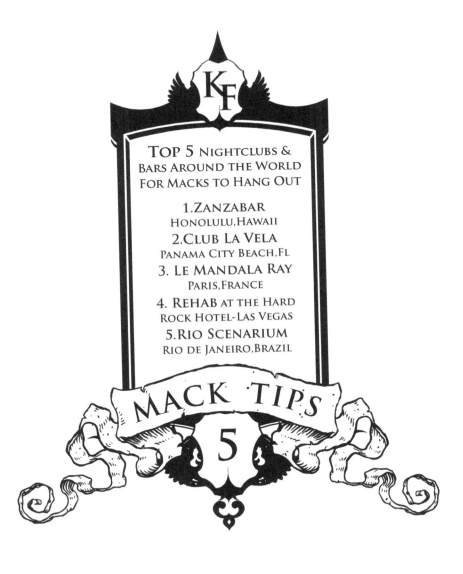

TOP 5 NIGHTCLUBS &
BARS AROUND THE WORLD
FOR MACKS TO HANG OUT

1. ZANZABAR
HONOLULU, HAWAII
2. CLUB LA VELA
PANAMA CITY BEACH, FL
3. LE MANDALA RAY
PARIS, FRANCE
4. REHAB AT THE HARD
ROCK HOTEL-LAS VEGAS
5. RIO SCENARIUM
RIO DE JANEIRO, BRAZIL

MACK TIPS

5

"Whosoever desires constant
success must change his conduct
with the times. "

— Niccolo Machiavelli —

Chapter Six

GUARANTEED WAYS TO GET SEX FROM WOMEN

It's 3:00 a.m. on a Saturday night. You've just pulled a female out of a club. You've convinced her to come home with you. Your game has been pretty strong up until this point, but now you feel stumped. You want to hit that ass, but you aren't sure how to approach the female about it. You think to yourself, "I don't want to be *too* forward, because she might get offended. And I don't want to appear overly anxious, because she might get turned off. I don't want to be overly aggressive, because I don't want to catch a case."

These are some of the thoughts that go through the minds of many guys when they find themselves in a compromising position with a female. In this chapter, I will give some tried and proven techniques that will help you talk a woman into giving it up more than willingly. I will also offer you precise rebuttals to every objection a woman may have to giving it up.

Even though these techniques can be used throughout the duration of your courtship with a female, they are best used on the first or second date. When you first hook up with a female, her expectations of you are much higher than when she has spent a little more time with you. In other words, she already has an idea of how she wants your relationship to turn out, so all you have to do is cater to her ideas and expectations. And the best way to do that is to not reveal too much of yourself at this point. You may be the nicest guy in the world, but in the back of her mind, she may be hoping that you are a thug. At this point she doesn't know that you are a really nice guy, but if it will help her give up the ass faster, let her think that you are a thug.

Getting Her to Your Crib

Let's say you've met a female at a club and you aren't able to pull her. You exchange numbers and play "phone tag" with one another, and now you two are trying to arrange a hookup. Since so many men come at females with the brown-nosing approach, many women are dying for a man to sort of put them in check, so to speak.

This doesn't mean to act rude or disrespectful when dealing with a female. What I'm saying is that a true mack should take control and bring closure to a situation, especially when that situation requires a decision (be it major or minor). You must remain in control of the decision-making, without coming off as a control freak. Now, let's say the female wants to come over to your crib and break you off a little something. In most cases, she's not going to come right out and say she wants to break you off. She wants to be macked into it. Since she doesn't want to come off as being too forward or too easy, she will often give *you* the opportunity to mack her into it. She often does this by making "decoy inquires."

An example of this is when a female wants to come over to your crib in the middle of the night, and she innocently asks you something like, "So, what are we going to do when I get there?" (knowing full well what she wants to do). Most brothers will respond to this by saying, "We're just going to talk," etc. The lack of creativity in this response often turns women off. Females will throw out a decoy inquiry such as this so that you can give her a reason to justify her coming over. If a female throws a decoy inquiry at you, don't ever act unsure or indecisive with your game. To females, this is a sign of weakness. Even if you don't want to respond to her "inquiries," you should still get your point across and bring closure to the situation. The conversation should go like this (while speaking over the phone):

Female: "So, what do you want to do tonight?"

Mack: "Well, you just come over here and we'll see what's crackin'."

Female: "Do you have anything planned? What are we going to do when I get over there?"

Mack: "Look, I'm a spontaneous dude, so let's just take care of A and B, then we'll worry about C and D."

Notice how the mack came across definitively and self-assured, without giving in to her decoy inquiry. This is also a very important screening process, because if a female really likes you (and doesn't have an alternative agenda), she will be content on just kickin' it with you, giving you both a chance to get to know each other. But if she is persistent on you two going out somewhere (like a restaurant, etc.), she may be an undercover chickenhead trying to mack up on a free meal.

The following mackin' techniques that I am going to discuss are designed to take place when you are in a compromising position with a female. You should have already followed the techniques in the other chapters to learn how to get a female in a position to get busy with you.

As I mentioned earlier, women know within the first few minutes of meeting a man whether she wants to have sex with him or not. All the man has to do is not mess it up. **But** most men *do* salt themselves, and the main reason they do is because they are thrown off by a woman's *objections.*

These guys have to realize that the average female they go out with on a first date is not just going to walk into their homes, bend over, and say "Okay, you can fuck me now." Although there are some females that are loose like that (trust me, I know), these types of incidents happen very rarely.

Therefore, you are going to have to use a little verbal persuasion to help get her out them draws. As I implied earlier, the main reason a female throws out these so-called "objections" (or decoy objections) is because she doesn't want to come across as being ho'ish or sexually undisciplined.

Basically, females want *you* to give them a reason to want to have sex with you. They want you to say something convincing, and they want you to say something that makes sense. They don't want to just give in to one of your lame lines, because they figure it will make them look easy. This is why it is important for you to be smooth and to say something sensible.

When in a compromising position with a female, it's not easy for a guy to try and make sense with a hard dick. This type of situation makes men say dumb things, and this in turn, causes men to resort to desperate measures and desperate approaches.

First of all, men have to understand that most females have heard all the lame lines that guys use while they are in compromising positions. Here are some examples:

Top 13 lame things men say to get sex from women:

1)."I love you" (**the bold face lie approach**).

2)."If you really cared about me, you would do it" (**the guilt trip approach**).

3)."Take off your clothes so I can give you a massage"(**the "I'm hooking *you* up" approach**).

4)."Let me just put the *head* in" (**the bargaining approach**).

5)."I normally don't have sex on the first date either, but you're special" (**the brown-nosing approach**).

6)."I'll buy you anything you want" (**the "tricking" approach**).

7)."I just *got* to have you"(**the "going for sympathy" approach**).

8)."There are a bunch of other girls that would love to do it with me" (**the "egotistical" approach**).

9)."I just wanna go down on you?" (**the "if I can't beat it, can I eat it" approach**)

10)."Okay, then just 'go down' on me" (**the Bill Clinton approach**).

11)."I just want to put it in, and take it right back out" (**the let me sample it approach**).

12)."Let's just take off our clothes. We don't have to do nothing" (**the take my word for it approach**).

13)."You want a ride home, don't you?" (**the hostage approach**).

These are the most common things that men say when they are trying to get sex, and here are some of the reasons why many of these lines don't work. By using the **boldface lie approach**, you immediately lose all of your creditability with the female. When you say things like, "I love you" or "I really want to be with you," and you haven't had a chance to get to know the female, she knows it's drama. Women often feel like men are insulting their intelligence if they think these lines are going to really work.

By using the **guilt trip approach**, men try to make females seem obligated to have sex with them, and this quickly kills the mood. When a female is in the mood for sex, she wants to do it within a comfortable scenario, and on her own terms. When a woman feels pressured, her defense mechanisms immediately go up, thus lessening your chance to hit it.

By using the **egotistical approach**, bragging about how many other women you can have, the first thing that comes to the female's mind is, "If you have so many other females that want to get with you, why aren't you with them?" Plus, the egotistical approach is just plain immature.

The **brown-nosing** and **tricking approaches** simply make you look desperate. The **going for sympathy approach** does work on certain females, because they may feel sorry for you, then decide to toss you a bone. But most females aren't down with giving up pity pussy, and using the going for sympathy approach will only get you tossed to the curb.

Sending the Right Vibes

When trying to get a female in the mood, it is very important that you send the right vibes. The problem with most brothers is that they often send off vibes that are obviously manipulative. And once a female has figured out your game, a lot of the intrigue is lost. Now the word *vibe* is very important in trying to get sex from females, and you should use it often. Since women are more emotionally driven than men are, they can relate more to a brother who is trying to build a good vibe with them. The very meaning of the word vibe (which is short for "vibration") is "an emotional aura that can instinctively be sensed."

It is commonly said that humans have five senses, when in reality we only have one, and that is the sense of touch (feel or vibration). The reason we have sight is because light *vibrates* the retina in our eyes and sends signals to the brain. The reason we "hear" is that sound *vibrates* our eardrums and sends signals to the brain, so on and so forth. Basically, all of our senses are based on certain vibrations, and women are more in tune with negative and positive vibes that others give off. In other words, a female usually knows when a brother is full of shit. So, when you're trying to" do something such as convince a woman to have sex with you, it's very important that *you* believe the game that you're kicking.

Overcoming Objections

As I stated earlier, when a man and woman are in "negotiations" to have their first sexual encounter with each other, the female will normally throw out a decoy objection to add a sense of adversity to the situation. It is important that a potential mack doesn't get thrown off course by her objections. He must have quick and precise rebuttals to her every objection so that he will stay on track.

Although every woman is different, I have learned that there are **six common objections that are used by most females**. These objections usually start off like:

"I would love to have sex with you, but..."

1)."I just met you, and we don't know each other well enough."

2)."I normally don't do it on the first date."

3)."Sex is important to me."

4)."If we have sex, that will change things."

5)."I have to be in love with a guy before we have sex."

6)."I just got out of a relationship and I'm not ready."

There are three "rebuttal levels" that you can use to overcome these objections. And, in using these three levels, you accomplish three things:

Rebuttal Level 1: You question her maturity.

Rebuttal Level 2: You minimize the significance of sex.

Rebuttal Level 3: You tell her what she wants to hear.

Now, before I go into depth about the rebuttals, there are other helpful tactics that you should be aware of. First of all, when using your rebuttals (once you're in a compromising position with a female), make sure you use the slow and low technique I described in the previous chapter. The more mellow you talk, the more relaxed the female will be. It's understandable that when the average man is sexually aroused, it's hard to be "mellow" in your demeanor. But, as a mack, you must understand the concept of mind over matter.

Also, when a female seems to have her defense mechanisms up, it's always helpful to get her in an *affirmative* frame of mind. One way of doing this is to get her to answer questions that she can only answer *yes* to. These are known as "common sense questions." This technique is commonly used by people who work in "sales." There's a saying that if you get a person to say "yes" five times, you have them sold. When a salesperson is pitching a product, and is about to close the deal, he will often use the "five common sense questions" technique on the buyer. This technique can be used in any situation, including a potential sexual encounter. Here are examples of a salesman trying to sell a product, and a mack trying to get up on some ass, by using the five yes's technique:

Salesman: "You're a smart person, right?"

Buyer: "Yes."

Salesman: "You want to do what's right for your business, right?"

Buyer: "Yes."

Salesman: "You like to be more cost effective?"

Buyer: "Yes."

Salesman: "You like to save money, right?"

Buyer: "Yes."

Salesman: "Well, if **I** can offer you a product that is better for your business, that is more cost-effective, and can save you money, that's something you would be interested in, right?"

Buyer: "Yes."

(Bam! He got the sale.)

Now here is the same technique used in a potential sexual encounter:

Mack: "You're a mature young lady, right?"

Female: "Yes."

Mack: "You know what's best for you and your happiness, right?"

Female: "Yes."

Mack: "You have a genuine interest in me, and you know I have a genuine interest in you, right?"

Female: "Yes."

Mack: And we have a good vibe going on so far, right?"

Female: "Yes."

Mack: "So, if a guy stepped to you that was better for you, that you had a genuine interest in, that had a genuine interest in you, and that had a good vibe going on with you, that's a guy you would wanna be down with, right?"

Female: "Yes."

(Bam! You got the draws.)

By asking a female these types of questions, you give her no choice but to be in agreement with you, because it would make her feel silly if she were to disagree. This is especially so when questioning a female's *maturity.* One thing that most women can't stand is being labeled as immature, and they will go to great lengths to prove their womanhood.

Also, when you are using rebuttals to overcome her objections, you have to make it seem like it's *her* decision to have sex. A female may become uncomfortable when she feels pressured in any way. And whatever you do, don't act as if you are desperate for the coochie. Grabbing, panting and pleading a woman for sex only makes you look like a buster.

The following rebuttals should be recited *verbatim* if you are not a seasoned mack. Once you've gotten the hang of the game, you can then spice it up with some of your own flavor. If you are in a compromising position with a female, and you recite these rebuttals word for word, your sex ratio is guaranteed to increase significantly. (It's also important to note that you should end each rebuttal by reiterating how well you two "vibe" together.)

If she says: "I would love to have sex with you, but ..." "I just met you, and we don't know each other well enough yet."

You say (using rebuttal level 3): "Look, (her name), let's say, hypothetically, we waited three months down the line to become intimate. If I'm an asshole now, I'm going to be an asshole three months from now. If I'm a great guy now, I'm still going to be a great guy three months from now. And I don't believe that you would be with me now if you didn't think I was a great guy. We have a good vibe going on right now, and we should continue that vibe."

If she says: "I have a rule that I normally don't do it on the first date."

You say (using rebuttal level 1): "I like a woman who is spontaneous. I don't like girls' who hold on to prerequisites about doing what they feel. I like a spontaneous woman, because spontaneity is a sign of maturity, and maturity in a woman is sexy to me. And a woman who is mature enough to do what she wants to do, when she wants to do it, is very sexy to me."

If she says: "Sex is important to me."

You say (using rebuttal level 2): "Y'know, people place too much emphasis on sex. The act of sex is as common and as natural as drinking water. Rabbits have sex. Ants have sex. Fleas have sex. Nearly every living species on the planet has sex, so sex shouldn't be used as a trump card in a relationship."

If she says: "If we have sex, that will change things."

You say (using rebuttal level 3): "A good relationship should be based on two people's ability to communicate, vibe and get along with each other mentally and spiritually. "Getting intimate" is just the icing on the cake."

If she says: "I have to be in love with a guy before I have sex."

You say (using rebuttal level 2): "Look, sex is not an accomplishment in a relationship. Maintaining a bond with your mate should be the main accomplishment, and "getting intimate" is just a *method to* maintain that bond. We have a good vibe going on right now, and we should continue that bond."

If she says: "I just got out of a relationship and I'm not ready yet."

You say (using rebuttal level 1): "You seem like a young lady who is mature enough to move on and not linger in the past. Now, I'm not saying this to try to convince you of anything. I just hope that you are mature enough to make decisions based on your own reasoning and expectations, and not on past hurts."

As I mentioned earlier, these rebuttals are guaranteed to work if you use them properly and in the right context. It's also important to note that when you are using these rebuttals, always give the impression that you are not trying to convince the female to have sex with you.

Always make it seem like you're speaking in a hypothetical sense. This is why it is so important to end each rebuttal with statements such as "We have a good vibe, and we should just let it flow" or "We should let our vibe flow naturally." Unless you are a seasoned mack, never make direct statements relating to the two of you having sex, such as "C'mon, let's do this" or "You know you wanna do it." This makes a female feel like you are pressuring her. So this is why it is important to keep your comments in a hypothetical context, because this makes the female feel like it's her decision to engage in "relations."

And, whatever you do, never, ever beg a female for the coochie. (This can get your T.M.A. membership revoked.) A man with game doesn't have to beg. Never give a female the impression that she's doing you a favor by giving you some. She will get as much pleasure out of the sexual act as you will. So, convey the message that this will be an experience you both will *share.*

Now, there are many instances where a female really doesn't want to do it, and you should take heed to these messages. These are the cases where no does mean no, and you should take the woman's word for it, and back up off that ass.

Here is a list of the top five objections women use when they *really* don't want to have sex (and the ones that you should take heed to):

1)."It's that time of the month."

2)."I have gas."

3)."The clinic results aren't back yet."

4)."1 don't feel 'fresh' down there."

5)."I need the money up front."

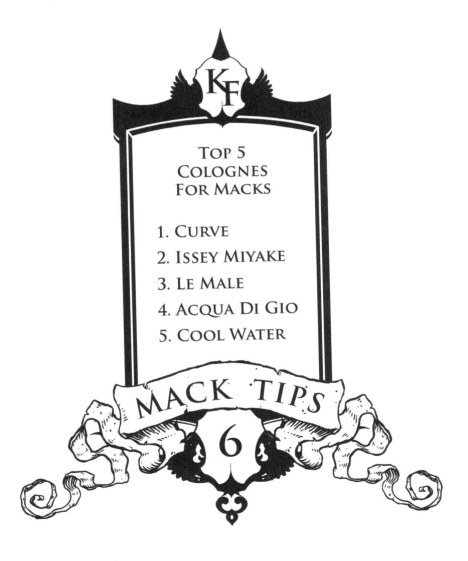

TOP 5
COLOGNES
FOR MACKS

1. CURVE
2. ISSEY MIYAKE
3. LE MALE
4. ACQUA DI GIO
5. COOL WATER

MACK TIPS

6

"Calm self-confidence is as far
from conceit as the desire to
earn a decent living is
remote from greed."

— Channing Pollock —

Chapter Seven
HOW TO BE A GIGOLO

Let's say you don't want to be a pimp, but you still want females to break you off a little paper every now and then. I'm going to show you how to obtain that goal. A gigolo is basically a "diet pimp," but his mackin' tactics aren't as extreme as a real pimp's. There is a thin line between a gigolo and a chili pimp. The general definition of a gigolo is a male who is paid to be an escort or a man who is supported by a woman. Historically, most *professional* gigolos work through reputable escort agencies that cater to a mostly white clientele.

Gigoloing was once considered strictly a white guy's game, because the only females who could afford to pay for play were older well-to-do white women, who were looking for young white studs. In modern times, there are more Black men getting into the gigolo game, professionally and independently.

As with any other aspect of the mackin' game, being a successful, independent gigolo depends on the females you choose. This also depends on how well you screen and qualify women. Trying to kick gigolo game to a broke chickenhead-type female is a waste of time; that's like trying to fish for a whale in a pond.

There are females that are just simply ineligible for this type of mackin' game. In order to get the big fish, you have to go to better waters. You have to look for females who are qualified to give you the paper that you feel you deserve. There are plenty of available, financially stable women who are just looking for a lil summ'in summ'in every now and then from a player. And, if your game is tight, you can be broken off (financially) handsomely for your services.

Don't Be a Mooch

It's important to note that there is a difference between a gigolo and a mooch. A gigolo is a player who has himself together, and when properly compensated, is willing to accommodate a female, on his own terms. A mooch is a guy who is just living off females. These types of men are also referred to as "niggalos," and they are in constant jeopardy of getting their T.M.A. membership revoked.

Although any one of the "4 P" guys could qualify as a niggalo, the "parolee" often occupies this category. Since most of the niggalo's clientele are hoodrats, ghetto queens, hoochie chickenheads, and low-budgets, he is also known as the "county check pimp."

The niggalo is totally content with collecting chump change from all of his ghetto girls on the first of the month. Another type of niggalo mooch is the "professional baby-daddy." This type of guy purposely has children by as many women as possible so he can have a reason to mooch off them. What the mooching brother doesn't understand is that you can only mooch for so long. When these needy types of men step to a female with the "*potential* pitch" ("I'm about to get a new job"; "I'm planning on going back to school"; "I'm about to get a record deal"; "I'm about to get drafted into the NBA") or a sad story ("I just can't find a job"; "I need money to go back to school"; "I just need a little help," etc.), this causes some women's maternal instincts to come out and then they want to nurture these brothers. Consequently, these women start to become mother figures to these men. These guys eventually become lazy, and they start to act as if they were these women's children. The mooching man will eventually move into the woman's home, and since he is living rent-free, he doesn't feel that he needs a job. He can kick it around her house all day (and if he's with a ghetto girl, he usually baby-sits her kids), playing video games, watching television, and waiting for the surrogate mother to come home and feed him. This type of dude has the nerve to think he's a mack. He doesn't realize that he can't "live off the tittie" forever. Once you become a mooch, the woman that you are mooching from will eventually get tired of you. Even the "mother bird" will kick the "baby bird" out of the nest sooner or later. And once a female realizes that you are not going to better yourself, you're going to be history.

To be a *gigolo,* you have to have your own thing going on. Even if you are solely dependent on a female for financial support, don't show it. At least, give her the impression that you are self-sufficient, and that you can do just fine without her.

Which Women to Go For

The best women to satisfy your gigolo agenda are the established or mature topnotch females. Although many middle-class females qualify, top-notch females are more financially eligible to satisfy your needs. From my experience, the best females to satisfy this agenda are single, mature females in the mid- 30's/early 40's age range, who still take good care of themselves. Top-notch women in this age group who are still single usually look years younger than they are, and they take great pride in their appearance.

Since many of these women have youthful appearances, younger men are often attracted to them. In most cases, when females are approaching their 30's, they start to focus heavily on "finding the right man to settle down with." They do this because society places a certain stigma on women who are in their 30's and not married. In many instances, when a woman feels that her biological clock is ticking, her standards will become lower and lower when rushing to find a mate, and she will end up just settling. Over the course of time, she will become content with the man she just settled for, and she will become more homely in her appearance.

In other words, when these females become comfortable within their relationships, they tend to let themselves go, and if their mates leave them for other women that are more well-kept, the homely woman will become bitter towards men from this point on.

Top-notch females, on the other hand, are on top of their game. Top-notch women in this age range are the sexiest of females, because they know how to keep themselves up and they know how to treat a man. They've played the "bitter role" and all the other relationship games before, and since that didn't work for them, they now act like they have some sense. Instead of becoming frustrated with men because of failed past relationships, they decide to focus more on their careers, and the less likely they are to lower their standards and just settle for any mate.

Many older men that are socially or financially capable of stepping to one of these mature, top-notch females are either already married or have no verbal skills. They often try to step to these women with offers of financial support, but these women are more than capable of supporting themselves. But these women *do* need a fella who can hit that ass right. That's where the *young mack* comes in.

Like most women, these women start to reach their sexual peak in their late 30's/early 40's. The only difference is that the top-notch women have the option to choose a young, vigorous stud to satisfy her sexual needs, and she is more than willing to hit him off with some paper to do so.

Rules of the Gigolo Game

Unlike the pimp game, where you're best advised not to have "relations" with your females, one rule is that the gigolo is going to have to tap that ass every now and then. In actuality, to turn a female out, so to speak, all you have to do is hit that ass one or two good times. The more anticipation you build up for you and your female to have another sexual experience, the more paper she will give you.

A good gigolo will have sexual relations with his female clients as little as possible. He has to let the females know that his time is valuable, and if they hook up to go to the movies, to dinner, to a play, or even to a hotel room, he has to be properly compensated .

Many people think gigolos manipulate and prey on unsuspecting older women, but this too is another mackin' myth. Most of the women that choose gigolos are married women who are not being satisfied by their husbands, career women who just want a boy toy for the weekends, or middle-aged females who just want a brother to make them feel young again. As long as both parties are straight up and honest about their intentions, there will be no need for deceit or wrongdoing.

The best way to deal with these women is to be very direct. Don't be afraid to crack them for some paper. However, if you try to *con* them out of money by telling them a bunch of bullshit, making up stories, or giving them the "potential pitch," they will lose respect for you, because they don't like to be played for the fool. So it's best when you tell them straight up "Look, before we go out, I need $300 to take care of some business" or "I gotta get this rent taken care of," etc. If you both have a true understanding of the game, she will be more than happy to oblige.

Here's a secret that most men aren't hip to. Most women would love to have a man that they can spend money on. I know that this may seem hard to believe because of the "chickenhead epidemic" that's going around. But you had best believe that if these chickenheads had the means to break their men off some paper, they would. If you ever hear a woman say, "I would never spend money on a man," I can almost guarantee that she doesn't have anything to give anyway. But a female who is financially stable has no problem with making the man in her life happy, even if she's not seriously committed to him. As long as he makes her feel good, she is going to do whatever she can to make him feel good.

As I mentioned earlier, the act of turning out a female is more of a mental game than anything else. This is especially so when dealing with women who have issues of insecurity and self-doubt. But turning out a female who is totally confident within herself relies on mental as well as sexual skills. When running your gigolo game on a mature, top-notch sista, you have to always maintain a position of control (socially and sexually). Since these women are so used to being aggressive and in control of their careers and social lives, many *average* brothers feel a sense of intimidation when dealing with them.

Essentially, these women have a secret desire for a brother to come along and put them in check. As a mack, you have to maintain a sense of mental and sexual dominance over these women. You have to take the initiative on when you and your female client will become intimate. You also have to take the initiative on how the sexual act will be played out. The fact that you are taking total control of the situation causes the woman to be mentally stimulated. There are also a few sexual tactics you can use to aid you in the act of turning her out. Although every woman has different "sexual needs," there are some sexual techniques you can use that are somewhat universal. These sexual techniques work best when used in conjunction with mental stimulation. (I will try to explain these techniques without being *too* explicit.)

How to Freak Your Female Gigolo Style

When making love gigolo style, you don't have to necessarily engage in any outrageous acts such as whips and chains or "handcuffs and blindfolds. Doing it gigolo style involves many simple, yet effective, maneuvers that will help the female reach her climax. One technique you can use is the "captured slave" technique. This is where you get on top of the female in the "missionary position" and hold her arms over her head while crossing her wrists (as if she were a captive). While holding her arms down in this position, you continue to get your stroke on. This causes her to feel a sense of submissiveness, and many women are turned on by this.

Another technique you can use is the "stick shift." This is where (while remaining in the missionary position) you place one of her legs into your forearm, and instead of pumping your hips back and forth, you pull your "member" out halfway, then move your hips from side to side, while slowly working your way back in. (Many women like the sensation that this technique causes on their "region.")

Another maneuver to use is the "press and grind" technique. This is where (while still laying on top of the female) you insert your member into her as deeply as possible, so that your groin is pressing up against hers. Then you grind on her clitoris as vigorously as possible until she reaches her climax.

There are also other, more creative ways to stimulate your female partner. One of my own inventions (and personal favorite) is a technique that I call the "tornado." Performing the tornado has a lot to do with psychological intrigue as well as sexual stimulation.

Now, this technique can be used by squares and macks alike, and it doesn't necessarily have to be performed on females who are "gigolo prospects." It can be performed on any female that you want to make a lasting sexual impression on. The tornado works best when it's performed on a couch, sofa or loveseat (so you should guide the female into the living room). In order to perform the tornado, you're going to need three things:

1).A towel

2).A glass of warm water

3).A box of strong breath mints (preferably Altoids)

It is important to note that the tornado is a technique you should "keep in your back pocket," so to speak, and save for a rainy day. You should do it every blue moon, because half the stimulation of it is that it is something different. By doing it on a regular basis, you will kill the novelty of it.

First, you have the female bring you the towel and the warm water. This alone will cause her to become intrigued, because now she's trying to figure out what you are about to do. You then have her remove her clothes. Next, place the towel on the sofa and have her sit down on it. (This will prevent the sofa from getting wet.) You then sit on the floor between her legs. Place a strong breath mint into your mouth and begin to perform "oral relations" on the female. The strength of the mint will give her vagina a cool, tingly sensation. This will cause her reflexes to tense up. After a few minutes of "minty cunnilingus," you then take a sip of the warm water and hold it in your mouth. Continue to perform oral relations on her while the warm water is flowing from your mouth onto her "vaginal region." The sensation of the warm water will cause her reflexes to involuntarily relax, thus initiating a climatic moment for her.

This technique is called the tornado because when the *cold* sensation collides with the *warm* sensation, it has the ability to cause much damage. And that's exactly what you're doing, tearin' up that coochie.

In the gigolo game, you must use techniques such as these as sexual secret weapons. They also can be used as bargaining tools to get your paper. You have to ration "skills" as if they were water, and when the female gets "thirsty" enough, she'll do whatever is necessary for a little "sip."

Here's a recap on ways to tell if you are a gigolo or a *niggalo*:

You are a Niggalo if...	But you are a Gigolo if...
1).You have to ask to borrow your female's car.	1).Your female breaks you off enough "cheddar" to buy your own car.
2).You have to baby-sit your female's kids.	2). Your female takes you and your kids on shopping sprees.
3).Your have to do whatever your female says, or she will put you out on your ass.	3). You call the shots with your female, and if she doesn't compensate you for your time, you can easily step to the next female who will.
4).Your females can't break you off paper until the first of the month.	4.) Your females hit you off with paper anytime you need it.

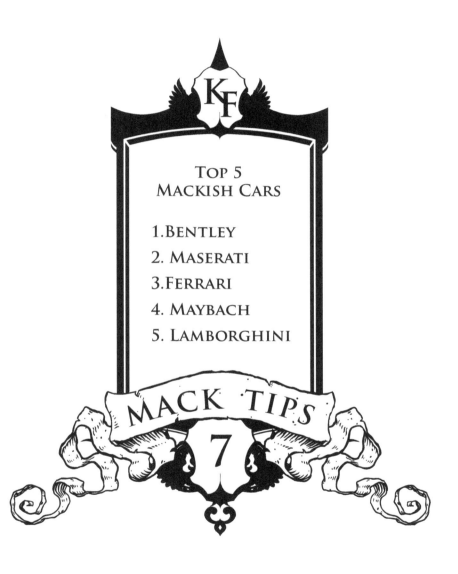

Top 5 Mackish Cars

1. Bentley
2. Maserati
3. Ferrari
4. Maybach
5. Lamborghini

MACK TIPS

7

"BEING ENTIRELY HONEST WITH ONESELF
IS A GOOD EXERCISE."

— SIGMUND FREUD —

Chapter Eight

HOW TO PEEP OUT GOLD DIGGERS

In the same way that we screen women for sex, many women also screen men to see if they are tricks. There are generally two types of females like this: the **needy wench** and the **gold digger**. Even though they may seem one and the same, these two females are as different as night and day. The needy wench usually falls into the hoodrat or chickenhead category, while the true gold digger, surprisingly, falls more into the top-notch category. Basically, the needy wench is a beggar, while the gold digger is a businesswoman.

One thing these two women *do* have in common is that they have no love for a true mack. A mack to these women is like kryptonite to Superman. These women generally seek out pushovers or professional guys. These women usually try to avoid macks because they know that a true mack can see through their game. When these women step to men, they have only one agenda in mind: to achieve financial or material gain.

Many guys often make the mistake of confusing the gold digger with the needy wench, and this causes them to get caught up. While the average guy is preoccupied with keeping his defenses up when dealing with a woman *he thinks* is a gold digger, a real gold digger is steadily milking his bank account dry.

The needy wench is more of a charity case than a gold digger. This is the kind of female that constantly begs a man until he finally tosses her a bone. This is no different from a homeless person standing on a corner with a cup in his hand, begging every pedestrian that walks by for change. If he begs long enough, eventually, someone will drop some spare change into his cup. This is what needy wenches do; they beg for little menial items.

Here are some examples of **things a needy wench will ask for (and what a real gold digger would never ask for) from a man:**

1). "Could you treat me to this new restaurant?"

2). "Could you get my hair and nails done?"

3). "Could you buy me this outfit?"

4). "Before you come by, could you stop and get me something to eat from McDonald's?"

5). "Can you pay my phone bill?"

When a needy wench screens through enough men, she's more than likely to run across a guy who will cater to her futile needs. But the results aren't nearly worth the effort. If you are going to do all that screening and running game on men, you need to be getting more than a Happy Meal.

A true gold digger understands this logic. This is why I actually have a lot of *respect* for a female who is a true gold digger. If a person has enough game to achieve their goals in a major way, I can't knock their hustle. A true gold digger is nothing but a "female mack." Also, the true gold digger is usually an extremely attractive female with a very impressionable personality. The thing I admire most about a true gold digger is that she is a real businesswoman. She understands that it takes money to make money, so she would never come across as being needy. A true gold digger would never beg a man for anything, because her game is so tight, she has men *offering* her what she needs.

Many needy wenches wish they had the type of skills a true gold digger has. Needy wenches often brag to their chickenhead friends about the little insignificant material items they obtain from men. You'll often hear them say things such as, "Girl, this nigga bought me this bracelet" or "Girl, I made this brother pay my gas bill," etc. Sadly, these women think they are doing major things by accomplishing minute goals. But, in reality, they are viewed as nothing more than bums.

The key to a gold digger's game is the way she defuses a man's defense mechanisms. The most common guy that a gold digger would normally step to is a man who would be considered a baller (a financially stable man). When a baller goes out with a female, automatically his defenses are up, because he knows that most of the women he dates are attracted to him because of his financial status. When he goes out with a female, he isn't sure if she likes him for him, or if she's trying to get something out of him, material-wise. And he, dealing with a number of needy wenches, only perpetuates his anxieties about dating certain women. The true golddigging female understands his paranoia, so she comes at him from a different angle. Instead of coming off as being needy, she shows him (or at least gives him the impression) that she is financially stable and content. She isn't openly impressed by his cars, jewelry or bank account, and she doesn't "ooh" or "ahh" over the guy if he has a fancy home or other extravagant material items.

One tactic that the gold-digging female will use on a baller when she first meets him is to take him out and pay for the entire date. By doing this, she gives the brother a reason to lower his defenses. This also gives the man the impression that she is not selfish. By her paying for the date, it also challenges his manhood. So, to prove to her that he is a "real man," he will reciprocate on a grander scale. He will go out of his way to show this woman (who he thinks is a regular top notch female) that he is appreciative of her. The more the gold digger offers to do things for the guy, the lower his defenses get. This, in turn, makes him feel a need to shower her with gifts.

Now, the average gold digger has at least three men that she is working in this manner. To an untrained eye, it can be very difficult to differentiate between the regular top-notch female and the true gold digger.

Here are three signs to look for which may suggest that a woman is a true gold digger:

1).**If she doesn't work, but she has a house full of fly stuff.** If it seems as if the female in question is always at home at any given moment during the day or night, that's a sign that she isn't employed full time. So, if you go to this seemingly unemployed female's home (and she claims that she lives alone) and she has expensive Italian furniture, valuable paintings, top-of-the-line electronic equipment, and Bentleys and Range Rovers parked in her garage, you may very well be dealing with a true gold digger, so be cautious. Sure, there may be other explanations for this type of female's upper-echelon lifestyle. She may sell weed on the low, low. Her baby's daddy may have been killed in a pit bull attack, and she's living off the insurance money. She may be selling pictures of her ass over the Internet. Or she could be a call girl. Who knows? Just approach the big-ballin' type female with caution, or *you* may be the next trick.

2).If she travels in and out of town on a regular basis. If your female in question is constantly saying things like, "I have to go to Vegas on Friday" or "I have to fly to New York on Tuesday to take care of some business," chances are she may well be a gold digger. Sure, there are women who have businesses and other legitimate reasons that may require them to travel in and out of town, but true gold diggers often have men flying them into different cities all around the country, so you have to peep game. The gold digger works best when her "victims" are not in the same city, so she has plenty of room to play. The gold digger also knows that it's hard for men to keep tabs on her when she lives in another city or state from them.

3).If she showers you with gifts, but doesn't want to give up sex. This is a classic example of a female mack's tactics. If a woman takes you out on the town every day for a whole week, spending money on you, and doesn't want to give up sex, this is almost a sure sign that this woman is a true gold digger. A lot of gold diggers like to play the sanctified, shy girl role, and come off as being the girl next door, but if the woman seems too good to be true, usually she is. The average man (not a true mack) can't see through the Ms. Goodie-two-shoes routine, and he ends up thinking that this girl may be the one for him.

And once he lowers his defenses, she goes in for the kill. If a woman is doing everything she can for a man, except having sex with him, she has one of two motives. Either she's, one, that rare breed of female that comes around once in a lifetime, who really wants to have a lasting emotional relationship. Or, two, she's a gold digger who is running game on a guy so that she can get some chips.

Peeping Out" Deceptiveness

There are signs in a female's behavior that will tell you right away if she's trying to be deceptive or not. Your ability to "peep" this behavior is essential for you to survive in the mackin' game. You either mack or get macked. One way to tell if a female is trying to be deceptive when you meet her is if she does an obvious "screen game" on you.

Here are some examples of the questions a potentially deceptive female might ask a man:

1). "So, how much do you make, doing what you do for a living?"

2). "What kind of car do you drive?"

3)."Who do you live with?"

It's important to note that the average true gold digger would never ask a man these types of questions, because she has other ways of screening a guy. She looks more into the way a man carries himself. Her goal is to get a baller, and she knows that most ballers don't walk around flashing all their wealth. She knows that a true baller is generally conservative, yet confident, and this is who she goes after.

But the average needy wench will ask the obvious screen game questions, and this shows that her game has no tact. Once you find out that a female is a needy wench, I suggest you move on to the next female who is feeling your swag. Wasting your time on a female like this is like trying to squeeze water from a rock. The reason it is so important to recognize these characteristics is that, if a female steps to you with deception, obviously she's trying to run some type of game on you to satisfy an ulterior motive.

Here are a few examples of deceptive comments and statements that some females make, and the translations of what they really mean:

If a female says:
"I'm a model, and I'm going to school" (when asked what her occupation is).

Translation:
This *really* means that she is broke, and she's trying to give you the impression that she is larger than what she really is. Just because a female has appeared in one hair show, this doesn't qualify her as a model. It's also a known fact that less than one percent (1%) of all *professional* models actually make a living at this line of work. So, if a female tells you she's a model, and her name isn't Tyra, Naomi or

Gisele, chances are she's an undercover needy wench who is trying to impress you with her so-called "credentials."

Although there are females that are going to school to get themselves together, a lot of irresponsible females are afraid to venture out into the real world, so they become "professional students." They use going to school as an excuse to just straddle along through life in limbo, while they live at home with their parents.

If a female says:
"I'm living back at home right now, because I'm helping my mama out" or "My mama is staying with *me* for a while" (when asked about her habitation status).

Translation:
This *really* means that she is still living at home with her parents, and the fact that she has to put a spin on the situation shows that she obviously has a complex about it. Don't get me wrong. There is nothing wrong with a person moving back in with their parents until they get themselves together, but at least be true to the game about it. If a person asks, just tell the truth and say, "I've moved back in with my moms'

until I get myself together, or until I save my money," etc. A man with an open mind will understand this completely. But if a female has reached a certain age, and she has *never* moved out of her parents' home, it's understandable why she would have a complex about it. A woman who stays at home with her parents is more prone to act immature and flaky than a woman who is living on her own.

When a woman has certain responsibilities in her life (such as paying rent and utility bills), she doesn't have time to bullshit around and play child-like games with men. A responsible female knows how to step to a player correctly.

If a female says:
"I'm an independent woman, and I don't need no man to do anything for me."

Translation:
If she says this, it **really** means that she *wants* to be an "independent woman," because if she were an independent woman, she wouldn't have to state it. It would just show through her actions. Women who make statements like this know that independence is what most men want in a female,

and these women are being somewhat deceptive, by simply stating what they think men want to hear. This is no different from a man saying to a woman, "I'm not like other men." Men say this because they think this is what women want to hear, but almost *every* man says it. You shouldn't have to *convince* people that you are a certain way, because it should already be evident. Could you imagine a woman like Oprah Winfrey running around bragging, "I'm an independent woman?" Absolutely not, because we can *see* that Oprah has paper like that. Your actions should always speak for themselves.

If a female says:

"I hardly ever go out..." (but you *met* her at a club, and every time you go out you see her in clubs).

Translation:

This form of deception speaks for itself because, obviously, the female is just straight up lying. If you meet a female with any of these characteristics, you should tighten up your game, and peep out her true motives. Another thing to look for when trying to peep out deceptiveness in a female is "deceptive flirting."

As I stated earlier, some women flirt with men strictly to get a positive reaction. These women feel they need to have a man pay special attention to them, so they can boost their own egos. Also, watch out for the sweet-talkers. If a woman is talking to you in a high-pitched, child-like, airy tone of voice, while batting her eyes, she may be preparing to run game.

There is also another type of female that is often mistaken for a gold digger. That female is the *groupie*. There are generally four types of groupies. Although these groupies have different names, they are basically all the same. They all want to get into lottery relationships by latching on to and living through successful people. **Here is a brief rundown of all four types of groupies:**

The Hip-Hop Groupie

Hip-hop groupies are usually Asian girls trying to pass for "hip," White girls trying to pass for Latinas, and Filipino girls trying to pass for Black. These females often frequent hip-hop clubs, sporting their expensive urban gear. You will often see these women wearing the baggy jeans, Timberland boots, hoodies and stocking caps. These females also know all the latest hip-hop dance steps and jargon.

The reason these groupies hang out at these spots is because upscale Black women generally don't go to strictly hip-hop clubs (especially in L.A.) on a regular basis. So these Asian, White, Filipino and Latina girls have all these Black men to themselves. These women take pride in bragging about how they dated somebody in the "Wu-tang Clan," or when they hung out with "50 Cent." And, if you don't have a record on the Top 10 rap charts, these women won't give you the time of day.

Since many of these females come from a fairly financially stable background, monetary gain is not their main agenda when dealing with brothers in the hip-hop community. One reason for this is the hip-hop music community is run by White boys, and despite the image of brothers rolling around in Benzos, poppin' bottles and rocking Rolexes, there is a very small percentage of brothers who are actually making any money in the rap game. (This is why many sistas can't afford to be strictly hip-hop groupies.)

There is nothing wrong with people from other races and cultures wanting to be down with the hip-hop generation, but you don't have to put up a front in order to do so. There are a few Country and Western artists that I personally like (such as Randy Travis and Garth Brooks). But you won't see me sporting a cowboy hat and some boots, driving a Dodge pickup truck, and talking in a Southern twang just to show my appreciation for their music.

Video Hoes

The video ho is also considered a "spot light freak." This type of female becomes a groupie because she thinks this may lead to her being discovered and becoming a star. These women have a good premise, but they often choose the wrong paths in order to obtain their goals.

Granted, you can achieve fame and fortune if you hook up with the right people, but these women often set their goals too low. Oftentimes, their main goal is to shake their asses in music videos.

This type of female only wants to sleep her way to the top of the music video world, and she is no stranger to the infamous casting couch. Instead of hooking up with a celebrity in order to achieve material gain (like a true gold digger would), all she wants to do is find out if she can appear in his next video.

The Backstage Pass Groupie

This type of groupie likes to hang out backstage at every concert that comes to her city. She normally has a female sidekick with her, and their goal is to sleep with as many members of a music group as possible. The fact that they can sleep with a celebrity gives them a sense of significance. This type of groupie is usually between the ages of 15 and 21. These young ladies are known to do just about anything, just so they can brag that they "did it" with "so and so." You will often hear these females say things like, "I dated two of the guys in G-Unit" or "I used to mess with three guys from Cash Money Records." In most cases, these females will grow out of the backstage pass groupie stage and square up, or they will graduate into a video ho.

Lakers Chasers

The sports groupie is the most extreme of the four types of groupies. The main goal for these women is to marry, or at least have a baby by, a professional athlete. The Lakers Chaser's whole life revolves around her trying to hook a sports star. It is unfortunate that so many of these women are so disillusioned to think that they can take the easy road through life by living off others and not bringing anything to the table. The odds of winning millions of dollars in the lottery are high, and the odds of meeting a multi-millionaire and living off him are just as high. So, just like it doesn't make sense for a person to sit around their home, being non-productive, while waiting for a lucky lottery number to hit, it also doesn't make sense for a broke female with no game to spend all of her time trying to hitch Kobe Bryant. These women are simply living off blind faith. Many of these women spend years "chasing the tour bus," and when they get older, they become bitter because they did all that chasing and have nothing to show for it. Plus, when a professional athlete *does* decide to get married, chances are it will not be to a broke female that came into his life after he made his millions. This is why most athletes end up marrying their high school or college sweethearts. The claim that all successful Black men want a White woman as a "trophy" is, for the most part, an inaccurate generalization (though there are many cases where this is true). People tend to date those who are equal to them socially. Unfortunately (or, fortunately, depending on your perspective), in this society many financially successful athletes feel they would have a better chance of finding a female that they can relate to, socially, in the White community. This is only because there are more White women in this country who come from more financially endowed backgrounds than Black women. So, in most cases, when a successful Black athlete does settle down with a sista, she is more likely to be a top-notch female who already has her shit together.

As I mentioned before, many groupies are often mistaken for gold diggers, but as with the needy wench, she too is only a decoy. The true gold digger is so cunning with her manipulative tactics, she can juice you without you ever knowing that you are being juiced. This isn't to say that you shouldn't keep an eye out for females who may be groupies or needy wenches, because if your game isn't at a certain level, you can get caught up by these women as well.

The Selfish Test

There are a couple of things to look for to determine whether or not a female is selfish. These little signs can help you see if the female is considerate, or if she thinks that the world revolves around her. The way a person acts on the first date usually sets the tone for the remainder of the relationship (if it even escalates into a relationship). Many people are already familiar with the "car door" test (as seen in the movie "A Bronx Tale"). This is when you are on a date with a female, and you open the door on the passenger side of your car to let her in. By the time you walk around to the driver's side of the car, you should look and see if she has unlocked the door for you from the inside. If she did unlock the door for you, this shows that she does have some form of consideration for others. If she did not unlock the door, this is a sign that she may be selfish and inconsiderate, and you should keep a leery eye on her.

Another way to tell if a female may be selfish or not is to go on a date with her, say, to a movie or to the theater, and see if she at least *offers* to pay half of the cost of admission. If you two walk up to the ticket counter and the counter person says, "That'll be $18.50," and your date opens her purse and says something like, "Are you straight?" or "How much do you need me to pay?" this shows that she does have some consideration. (In most cases, the man will decline her assistance.) But if the counter person tells you the price of the tickets and your date just stands there twiddling her thumbs, she may be a candidate for selfishness. (It is also important to note that, in most cases, a female who is genuinely considerate will at least offer to buy the concessions at the movies if she did not offer to pay for her ticket.)

Also, if you take a female to a restaurant and she eats damn near everything on the menu, and doesn't offer to pay half the bill, or at least leave the tip, she is a prime candidate for a selfish needy wench.

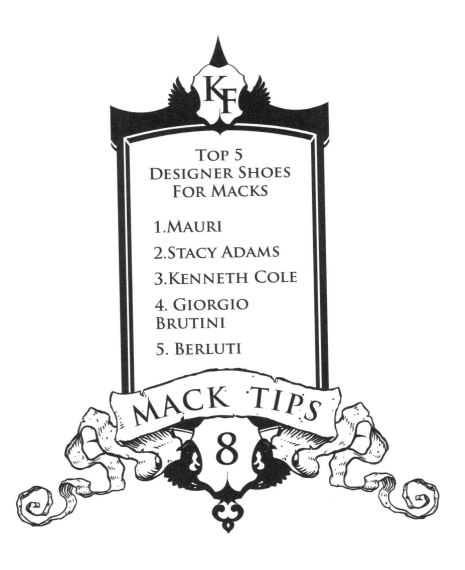

Top 5 Designer Shoes For Macks

1. MAURI
2. STACY ADAMS
3. KENNETH COLE
4. GIORGIO BRUTINI
5. BERLUTI

MACK TIPS

8

CONCLUSION

Now that I have hit you off with all this game, I hope you use your mackin' powers for good, not evil. Any buster can lie, deceive and *sneak* around with different women, but this doesn't require any type of game. A true mack is man enough to put everything out on the table and be very up front with the women he deals with. He's not afraid of the repercussions, because he knows that if one female isn't cooperative, the next one will be.

Remember that being a mack doesn't imply anything that is negative. A mack is just a man who knows the right thing to say, at the right time, in order to satisfy his agenda. Boxing promoter Don King is a perfect example of a mack. Don King has been an underdog in the media since the beginning of his career, and whenever people try to indict him on charges, accuse him of fixing a fight, or simply try to back him into a corner, he always has some type of clever response to mack his way out of the situation. President Obama is another example of a mack.He was a brother with humble beginnings who macked his way into the White House.

As I mentioned before, there is a difference between a mack and a player, and you should always try to elevate yourself to mack status. Even though being a player has its benefits, there are a few downsides of the "playing game." Since being a player has so many shortterm effects, unless you have a lot of time on your hands, the outcome usually isn't worth the effort. The smooth and suave demeanor of the player usually puts women in a semi-hypnotic state, and you have to move in fast in order to satisfy your agenda; it is only a matter of time before the female snaps out of it. Most females know that a player is just kickin' game, but many times she wants to hear his game anyway, because it puts her in a mild state of euphoria. However, this only lasts for so long, and once she snaps out of it, and reality kicks in, she usually gets mad at herself (and, subsequently, at the player) for falling for his game. This is why a player has to keep recruiting females.

Another downside to being a player is that you always have to be "on." Donning your player persona 24 hours a day can be frustrating, because when the real you finally does surface, you are unsure if your female cohorts will accept the real you or not. Since a mack is right there in between the player and the pimp, he has the option to swing to either side whenever it is convenient. And he can do this without losing his true identity.

There is a saying in the hustling community that a player is *made* but a pimp is *born*. All men have mackin' potential, but a true mack has to be groomed to perfection. Since the true mack inherits all the positive traits from all of the 4 P's, the mack is the closest thing to that perfect universal renaissance man that most women claim they're looking for. In all fairness, no one can technically be considered perfect, because everyone has a different criterion of what is considered perfection. To a crackhead man, his perfect woman would be a crack-ho. The perfect man for a woman into archeology is a man who is also into archeology. Since a mack is considered a top-notch male, the perfect female for him would most likely be a top-notch female.

So, as a mack, you should always set your goals and standards high. The problem that most women have is they want the proverbial perfect man (a true mack), but they are unable to keep and maintain that man once they get him. Every woman can *get* a man, but not every woman can *keep* him. Many people claim that they want certain things, but in reality, they are just not ready for them.

Many people claim that they want to own a Ferrari. But can they maintain the monthly payments? If the Ferarri breaks down, can they afford the expensive repairs that are needed? In most cases, the answer is no, because many people are not financially ready to maintain a car of that caliber. This is why people should have *themselves* together enough to maintain the things they aspire for.

As I mentioned earlier, the ideal female for a mack to deal with is a top-notch or middleclass female. Universally, the middle-class female is the most desired by men, because she is generally easy going and better to deal with. Also, remember that it is important for a mack to keep at least two very attractive, platonic female friends that he can go out and kick it with. When other women see you out with an attractive female, this sparks interest and intrigue. And, because of the competitive nature that many women have with each other, this makes other females want to see what you are about.

Another thing to remember is to never try to square up a ho (i.e. "turn a ho into a housewife") because hoes, like every other woman, have a need to satisfy all three of the relationship agendas (emotional, sexual and financial gratification). This is why hoes only deal with tricks, pimps and other hoes: Tricks give hoes financial and sexual gratification; pimps and other hoes give them emotional gratification. For all the guys that are trying to maintain their T.M.A. memberships, I have a list of the seven penalties that will cause your membership to be revoked. Remember, when you become a member of the T.M.A., you automatically get credited 10 points. Once your "mackin' mistakes" have deducted those points, you are no longer considered a mack, and you should just live your square life happily ever after.

Granted, everyone is entitled to make mistakes in life; this is how you learn right from wrong. However, it is how you rectify the mistakes in your life that determines your character. If someone asks you, "What is two plus two?" and you say "five," that's a mistake. But if someone shows you the correct answer, and you still insist the answer is five, then you are a legitimate fool. In the same way, if you are a man that is getting played by a female, and you don't utilize your option to rectify the situation with correct game, and insist on letting the female continue to play you, then you too are a legitimate fool. And you don't deserve the honor of being a T.M.A. member.

Seven penalties that will cause your T.M.A. membership to be revoked:

1). Paying a car note or utility bill for a female who is not your girlfriend or significant other (also known as "saving hoes") (*deduct 3 points*).

2). Fighting another man over a female if she chooses him (*deduct 3 points*).

3). Begging a woman for sex (*deduct 2 points*).

4). Stalking a female (*deduct 2 points*).

5). Lying on your dick (*deduct 2 points*).

6). Crying over a female because she might leave you (*deduct 2 points*).

7). Paying for sex (*deduct 5 points*).

People always ask me, "King Flex, since you are an expert on the art of mackin', what type of females do *you* like?" The following will give you some insight on my *personal* tastes, likes and dislikes about women. This will also give you an idea of what other true macks look for in women.

First of all, I prefer women between the ages of 21 and 34. I think most women learn to make more mature decisions around the age of 23. Plus, at this age many women start branching out on their own and becoming more independent. I have found that women who live on their own are much more mature than females who still live at home with their parents. As I mentioned earlier, the responsibility of living independently makes a person more mature, which in turn, makes them less likely to act flaky, less likely to bullshit and less likely to jive around when dealing with others. This is also why I don't like women who are professional students (as I mentioned in Chapter 8).

Most men have a unique *fetish* abut women that they like. To me, women with bow legs are sexy. And even though it is becoming somewhat of a cliche with men, I am also into nice feet on a female. To help give you an idea of what I like, physically and personality-wise, about females, here is a list of **five celebrity females that would be considered my type**:

1).**Halle Berry:** Not only does she have naturally cute looks, she has a very sophisticated vibe about herself.

2).**Stacy Dash:** This is a slim, brown-skinned honey, with bowlegs and a nice frame. She also has the same down-to-earth, middle-class girl persona that Halle Berry has.

3).**Eva Mendes:** (Cuban-American actress): This exotic latina has a lot of sex appeal that I find very attractive.

4).**Roselyn Sanchez:** (Puerto Rican actress): This is another spicey latina with all around sex appeal

5).**Beyonce:** Beyonce seems as if she was once a middle class girl who graduated to top notch status. Her round-the-way-girl aura is a perfect balance for her model good looks.

If I were able to build a female from scratch, her "build" would consist of the following:

She would have:

Halle Berry's *face*

Christina Milian's *hair*

Tyra Banks' *breasts*

Ciara's *stomach*

Kim Kardashian's *ass*

Charlize Theron's *legs*

Alicia Keyes' *feet*

Oprah Winfrey's *bank account*

Although I like a female who stays current when it comes to fashion, I do not like a female who is *trendy*. Most women that are into the latest trends usually tend to be followers, and I like a female who has leadership qualities. Living in a city such as Los Angeles, one is used to seeing females who torture and mutilate themselves (via implants, plastic surgery, liposuction, etc.) in order to look like the females in the latest magazines. Unfortunately, the *images* of women who grace magazine covers oftentimes set the standard of what a beautiful woman should look like. But, in reality, it's almost impossible for the average female to make herself look like the models in the magazines, because most of the models themselves don't even look like that in real life. These models have professional lighting, makeup artists, airbrush artists, etc. to help give them that "flawless look." The magazines also have computer generations that will remove any wrinkle, stretch mark, pimple, or any other natural quality that may be considered undesirable, from these print models. So, basically, the images of these models are not even real, and trying to emulate something that is not even real is insane.

Speaking of trends, another thing I am not too crazy about in women is ***trendy bisexuality.*** In the past few years, a lot of females have been riding the bisexual band wagon, and swinging both ways is now the thing to do. Now, understand, I do not have a problem with **lesbians,** but I do have a problem with some trendy bisexual women. There is a difference between lesbians, dykes and bisexuals. A **lesbian** is a regular, everyday woman, who just happens to exclusively date other females. I don't have a problem with that. A **dyke** is a female that is trying to be a man, and she too only dates other women. I don't have a problem with that either. But the trendy bisexual female is generally a toss up: She is usually down with whatever with whomever ,and she is usually an attention whore.. Unlike the **lesbian** and the *dyke,* who usually maintain a monogamous relationship with their partners, the trendy bisexual female is a borderline stank ho.

Although I, like most men, like a woman that is open-minded and sexually uninhibited, I do not like a female who is sexually *undisciplined.* Although I think it is important for a female to retain sexual *options,* it is equally important for her to have sexual boundaries as well. Another thing I personally am not too particularly fond of is a woman who *smokes.* Aside from giving females that masculine, raspy, phlegm-filled voice, and that tired, worn out, physical appearance, cigarette smoking also has implications of mental and psychological issues. Smoking, with some women, is a result of an oral fixation left over from childhood. Oftentimes when a child becomes agitated, he/she needs to have something in his/her mouth (a pacifier, a bottle, a nipple, a thumb, etc.) to feel secure. And, in many cases, people carry this regressive behavior into adulthood. So, whenever they have a problem or whenever they feel insecure, they pop a cigarette into their mouths for comfort. People who really don't know how to properly deal with their issues have even more extreme oral fixations. Whenever they get depressed, they will put a whisky bottle in their mouths. Whenever they feel lonely, they will stuff food into their mouths. Whenever they get confused, they will go so far as to put a crack pipe in their mouths. The point is that I tend to be weary of females with symptoms of having a regressive oral fixation, because this implies that she may not be able to correctly handle certain issues that come up in her life.

I do not want it to seem that I am putting too many expectations on women. From reading the previous pages, one might assume that I expect a female to be some sort of

Super Woman. The only thing that I *personally* expect from females is for them to possess **normal behavior,** and what is **normal** is not necessarily **popular.** Smoking is popular, but it is not normal. Plastic surgery is **popular,** but it is not **normal.** Being a slacker is popular, but it is not normal. Trendy bisexuality is popular, but it is not normal. This is why I prefer women who are leaders to women who are trendy: A **trendy** female will do what is popular, whereas a **leader** will do what is best for her. Since men are simple creatures, it does not take much to satisfy us. To keep us satisfied, all a woman has to do is apply the 3 F's:

Feed us

Fuck us

Finesse us

Many women feel that they have to go all out and be on some freak vibe in order to get a man's attention. But once the novelty of her freakishness wears off, a man wants to know if she can apply the 3 F's. Most women can only provide two F's at any given time, but if she can learn to apply **all** of the 3 F's, she should have no problems with the man in her life. If the aspiring macks out there maintain the positive characteristics of the 4 P's, they should have no problems with the females in their lives. And always remember: ***Be true to the game, and the game will be true to you.***

THE END

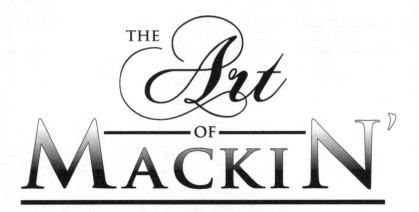

TARIQ "K-FLEX NASHEED
PRESENTS

A
SNEAK PREVIEW OF THE
FORTHCOMING NOVEL

"THE GAME ADVISOR"

I'm at the club,chillin' with my regular partners in crime. It's a usual Sunday night here in Los Angeles. Even though the club is packed, I'm still somewhat bored. I've been in the club a million times before, talked to most of the women in there; so nothing is really interesting me right now.

I'm sweating like a pig. The club feels like a sauna,and it doesn't help that I'm wearing this hot ass suit jacket. I'm wiping my face off with napkins, and the ones I've been using all night have soaked through. And I'm thinking to myself, *I need to go to the bar to get some more napkins.*

As I'm walking to the bar, a very sexy, sophisticated, brown-skinned cutie catches my eye — we catch each other's eye — for a quick second. I walk over to the bar, I grab some napkins, and I'm peeping her out. I have never seen her in this spot before. I'm thinking to myself, *I'm about to go over here and put some game down on her.*

So I walk over to her, and before I can say anything, she says to me, "Your face is fluorescent."

For a second, I'm thinking, *What the hell is she talking about?*

Then she says, "Your face. You have lint from your napkins all over your face, and the lights in the club are making your face glow."

I'm slightly embarrassed for a quick moment, but I regain my composure and I say, "OK, good lookin' out."

She then takes the fresh napkins out of my hand and starts wiping my face off for me.

"Let me help you out", she says.

I'm impressed so far.

It's very rare that a woman can throw me off my game; even a little bit.

So we make small talk, we chop up game. I find out her name is Tiffany, and she works at an investment firm in Beverly Hills. This woman is very unlike all the other women that I'm used to dealing with in Los Angeles. She doesn't have the L.A. glamour girl look, but she's extremely cute, very wifey-type material.

So I'm spittin' game at her, and I start going into my "Let's go to breakfast" routine, the infamous routine that I've used dozens of times on other girls to get them to leave the club and go home with me.

This young lady, Tiffany, had sparked a new flame in me. There was something about her vibe that I liked. And I've gotten girls out of the club dozens of times using the "breakfast" routine. Little do I know that this would be the last time I would want to use that routine and pull a girl out of a club for a one-night stand again.

Tiffany and I are making small talk, and I go in for the close.

I tell her, "Look, you and I, we're gonna go to breakfast tonight. I want you to meet me over at the door at 1:30, and then we're gonna get up outta here."

She says, "OK. That sounds like a plan."

So I walk back over to my entourage who now has a table in the v.i.p. section. They are rotating girls back and forth from our table all night. But I'm not paying too much attention to them. I'm just waiting on 1:30 to roll around.

I mingle with friends and associates, and at around 1:28, I look over at the door. Tiffany's standing by the door.

I'm thinking to myself, *Perfect.*

So I go over there to her. I say, "Alright, let's roll."

We go outside; she says, "Where'd you park?"

I said, "I valeted my car."

She said, "OK, I parked around the corner. I'm gonna pull around and you can follow me. I live in Redondo Beach."

I'm thinking to myself, *Perfect. She already knows*

what's up. This is easier than I though it was gonna be.

I get my car from the valet. I see her car; she has a white BMW.

I'm even more impressed.

I followed her. We take the 10 freeway to the 405 south, and we exit Crenshaw Blv.

For a split second, seeing Crenshaw Blv. made me a little concerned. I thought to myself *I hope this girl don't really live in the hood.* But I felt a sigh of relief when she made a right turn on 190th.

We pull up to her condo — ballin'. She had a real nice spot that was a block away from the beach.

I'm even more impressed.

So we go inside. It's immaculate. The furniture is tight, the decoration is tight, the carpet, plush. Everything is real upscale. I haven't been impressed by a woman like this in a long time. Tiffany was definitely wifey material. Very sexy young lady, very conservative, and I found that very attractive.

I'm peepin' out the crib, and she says, "Let's go upstairs."

So we go upstairs. The bedroom is tight — big, king-sized bed with a lot of satin pillows. The room is just real sexy and sensual. She puts on some music, and she turns on a red lava lamp; now the whole ambience of the room is real erotic.

She says, "Make yourself comfortable. Do you want anything to drink?"

I said, "Yeah, lemme get some juice. Do you have any juice?"

She said, "Yeah, I've got cranberry juice."

So she goes to get me some juice. I'm laying in the bed. I get comfortable, listening to the music she put on. It's was "The Best Of Sade" cd.

This girl was smooth.

I'm feeling the ambience of the room, vibin', really tripping on how fly this chick is. This woman is 26 years old, has a nice, square job, nice ride, nice crib, no kids. I don't even like square women like that, but if I do get with a square chick, *she's* the one.

She comes back upstairs with my beverage and says, "Lemme get these sweaty club clothes off and go shower up."

She goes in the bathroom, does her thing. I'm sitting up in the bedroom chillin', looking around at everything, very impressed, thinking to myself, *Man, I might have to give up all my other girls and make her The One.* I was that taken by this chick. I haven't met a young lady in L.A. who was this tight,who all around had it together like this girl did.

So she comes out of the shower. She has on panties and a tank top, and her body is more bangin' than I imagined. That was even sexier to me, because she had all that fine body hidden under those conservative clothes at the club.

I'm thinking to myself, *I'm about to knock the bottom out this ass.*

She walks seductively across the room and gets in the bed with me. We're chillin', still got the Sade music going, still got the lava lamp beaming.

I get up and say, "Hey, lemme go and freshen up a little bit because I'm still a little sweaty from the club myself."

I want to bring my "A" game to this girl tonight.

So I go in the bathroom. I find some baby wipes, and I wipe myself down a little bit, wash off all my essential parts, and just freshen up.

And I'm thinking to myself, *When I go in there, should I position the condom so I can have easy access to it?* But then I start thinking to myself, *You know what, this girl is so fly, I might not even need a condom. I might hit that ass raw dog.*

I mean, all these thoughts are going through my mind. She's so fly to me, I'm just throwing all types of judgment out the window.

But I think to myself, *Well, we'll see. I'll just play it out and see how things go.*

I freshen up and I'm now in my boxers and my t-shirt. I go back in the bedroom, ready to go in here and do my thing. I didn't notice how dark the room was until I got out of the bathroom. I'm trying to be cool but I'm trying not to bump into anything because I could barely see in front of me . The lava lamp is making the room look like our own little private club.

I walk over to the bed, and I look down at her, and it looked like what appeared to be tears going down her face. At first,I thought that my vision was just trippin' because it was so dark in the room.

But then I heard her sniffling a little.

I'm thinking to myself, *Damn, what's going on with this chick?*

Now I'm trying to think, *OK, lemme keep my composure. Lemme not get thrown off.*

I asked, "Hey, what's wrong with you? Everything alright?"

She was like, "Yeah, everything is cool. Everything is alright."

I'm thinking to myself, *Wow, I've never had this happen before.*

I've never had a female cry before sex, but as a mack and as a game advisor, you gotta be prepared for any kind of obstacles or road blocks that comes your way.

So anyway, I'm getting my mind prepared to have a good comeback to anything that's going on in this woman's mind. I'm just getting myself psychologically prepared to come back at her with some good game. Because no matter what she says, I'm gonna really spit some fly shit and sidestep whatever's bothering her ,and get her back in a comfort zone, so I can at least hit this ass tonight.

I say to her again,with a very concerned and nurturing tone in my voice, "Look, Tiff, what's going on with you, babe? You're crying, talk to me. What's going on with you?"

So, she wipes her eyes off, she clears her throat, and she sits up in the bed.

She says, "Well, I have something to tell you."

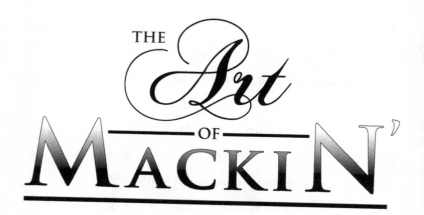

ABOUT THE AUTHOR

TARIQ "KING FLEX" NASHEED is an author/lecturer and television personality who has appeared on TV shows such as The Tonight Show with Jay Leno, Late Night with Conan,and several shows for MTV and VH1. He is also the host of the critically acclaimed Mack Lessons Radio Show (macklessonsradio.com). Tariq does lectures all around the country teaching men and women his strategies and techniques on dating and relationships. Tariq lives in Los Angeles,Ca.

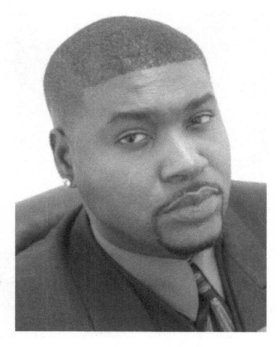

CONTACT INFO FOR KING FLEX:
KFLEX4LIFE@YAHOO.COM

WWW.MACKLESSONS.COM
WWW.MACKLESSONSRADIO.COM
WWW.KINGFLEX.TV
WWW.MYSPACE.COM/TARIQ_NASHEED
WWW.THEARTOFMACKIN.COM
WWW.THEARTOFGOLDDIGGING.COM

OTHER BOOKS BY
TARIQ "KING FLEX" NASHEED:

*THE MACK WITHIN
(PENGUIN)

* PLAY OR BE PLAYED
(SIMON AND SCHUSTER)

* THE ART OF GOLD DIGGING
(G.D. PUBLISHING - KING FLEX ENT)

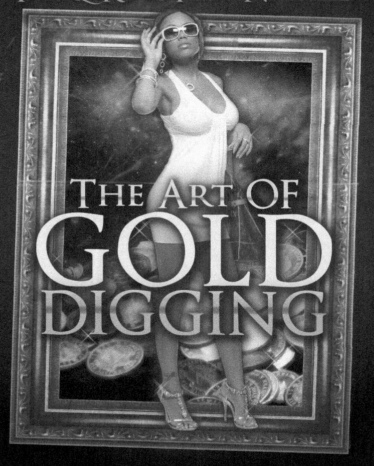

THE ART OF GOLD DIGGING

184 pages

Publisher. G.D Publishing-King Flex Ent.

The Art Of Gold Digging is the ultimate instructional guide to help women upgrade their game when it comes to dating. New York times best selling author Tariq King Flex Nasheed teaches women how and where to meet wealthy men and how to get these men to lavish them with gifts and riches.

THE MACK WITHIN

The Holy Book of Game

Tariq "K-Flex" Nasheed

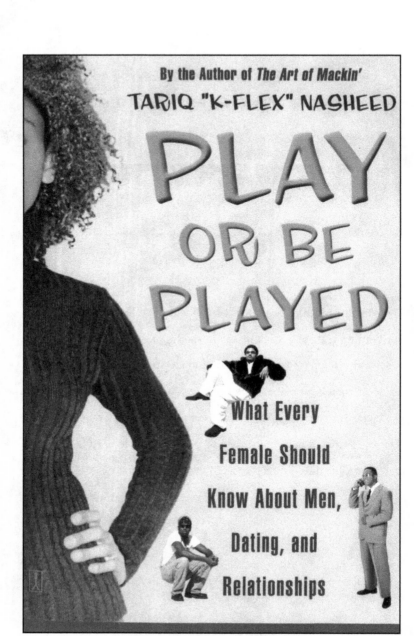

By the Author of *The Art of Mackin'*

TARIQ "K-FLEX" NASHEED

PLAY
OR BE
PLAYED

What Every
Female Should
Know About Men,
Dating, and
Relationships

Got Game?

It's a fact. Every woman needs game. Take Oprah, Jada Pinkett-Smith, and Beyoncé Knowles. All three of these women have the one intangible quality that every mack, male or female, must possess: they all have game. In other words, they have intelligence, hustle, and common sense that they apply to every aspect of their lives -- especially in their relationships.

Play or Be Played is an instruction manual for women who are tired of being played by men and who want to be players themselves. Though women may not want to play games, the truth is men often do. So women who hope to win in the game of love must first learn the rules. Bestselling author and true mack, Tariq "K-Flex" Nasheed shares:

ways to spot a scrub
what it takes to get with a baller
why men cheat
how men really judge women
the top three mistakes women make in relationships
Street-smart and straightforward, Play or Be Played will help you get with a king without being a hoochie, groupie, or a chickenhead.

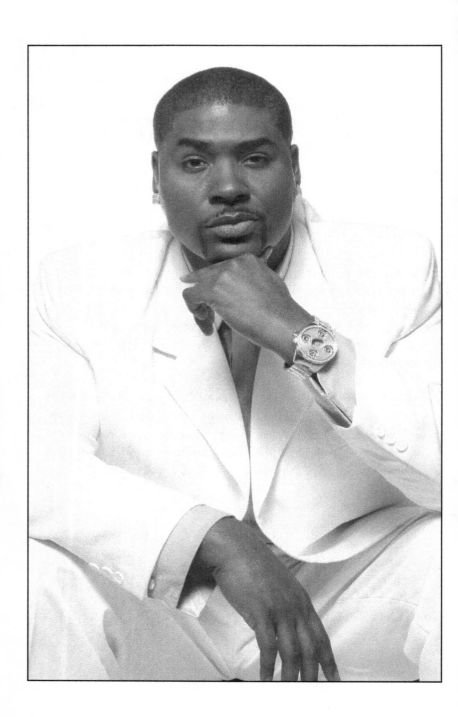

COMING SOON:

THE FIRST NOVEL FROM
TARIQ "KING FLEX" NASHEED

THE GAME ADVISOR

Based on a true story.

COMING

SUMMER 2009!

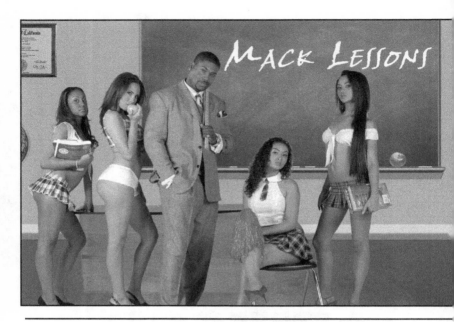